SPEEDRUNNER

SPEEDRUNNER

4 WEEKS TO
YOUR FASTEST LEG SPEED
IN ANY SPORT

PETE MAGILL

CONTRIBUTORS

Diana Hernandez, Sean Magill, and Eric Dixon

Boulder, Colorado

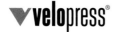 velopress®

3002 Sterling Circle, Suite 100
Boulder, CO 80301-2338 USA

VeloPress is the leading publisher of books on endurance sports. Focused on cycling, triathlon, running, swimming, and nutrition/diet, VeloPress books help athletes achieve their goals of going faster and farther. Preview books and contact us at velopress.com.

Distributed in the United States and Canada by Ingram Publisher Services

Library of Congress Cataloging-in-Publication Data

Name: Magill, Pete, author.
Title: Speedrunner: 4 weeks to your fastest leg speed in any sport / Pete Magill.
Other titles: Speed runner
Description: Boulder, CO: VeloPress, 2018. | Includes bibliographical
    references and index. |
Identifiers: LCCN 2017061627 (print) | LCCN 2018000735 (ebook) |
    ISBN 9781937716998 | ISBN 9781937715786 (pbk.: alk. paper)
Subjects: LCSH: Running speed—Handbooks, manuals, etc. |
    Running—Training—Handbooks, manuals, etc. | Running—Physiological
    aspects—Handbooks, manuals, etc. | Runners (Sports)—Handbooks, manuals, etc.
Classification: LCC GV1061.5 (ebook) | LCC GV1061.5 .M238 2018 (print) |
    DDC 613.7/172—dc23
LC record available at https://lccn.loc.gov/2017061627

This paper meets the requirements of ANSI/NISO Z39.48-1992 (Permanence of Paper).

Photos by **Diana Hernandez**
Art direction by **Vicki Hopewell**
Cover design by **Kevin Roberson**

18 19 20 / 10 9 8 7 6 5 4 3 2 1

CONTENTS

1

THIS IS SPEEDRUNNER

In sports, the difference between a star and an also-ran is tenths of a second.

Athletes who are faster, stronger, and quicker dominate. Athletes who lack these characteristics languish. This is true no matter the sport. In football, 40-yard-dash times can determine who gets playing time and who rides the bench. In soccer, the ability to execute a change-of-direction dribble can make the difference between a shot on goal or the defender clearing the ball. In basketball, there is no fast break on a team with slow feet. In tennis (which averages 3 to 5 changes of direction for 8 to 12 yards of movement per point), a sluggish first step can lead to a win—for your opponent. In baseball, your speed to first base can earn you a hit, while a middle fielder's speed and lateral quickness can rob you of the same. In volleyball, there's no spike or block without the vertical explosiveness to rise above the net. And in track & field, athletes who can generate the most horizontal and vertical force go home with the medals.

⟩⟩ SPEEDRUNNER

A student of advanced human locomotion; someone who trains his or her nervous system and muscles to produce maximum speed, power, and agility

In sport after sport, it's the speed, strength, and agility you produce with your legs that determines what you can accomplish on the field, court, or track.

There's an old-school saying in track & field: "God makes sprinters, coaches make milers." This outdated belief stems from the erroneous assumption that you're stuck with the speed that God, evolution, and your parents gave you. Maybe you can build a bigger heart and better endurance to become a miler, but improve your speed? *No way!* Except that modern sprint coaches figured out a way, and in 2016, a total of 23 runners recorded 53 performances at 100 meters that were faster than Carl Lewis (*Sports Illustrated*'s Olympian of the Century) ran for his 100-meter gold medal at the 1984 Los Angeles Olympics.

Across all sports, athletes are getting better, and their skill set of speed, strength, and agility is improving. When you consider that, in America, approximately 45 million youth athletes (ages 6 to 17) and 25 percent of the adult population are active in sports, coaches can be forgiven for skipping over athletes who aren't prepared. Frankly, if your skill set is lacking, you need to improve it. These days, showing up for a team-sports tryout or competition without a developed skill set is like taking on Joey Chestnut at Nathan's Famous International Hot Dog Eating Contest without an appetite.

Al Davis, the late, outspoken owner of professional football's Oakland (soon to be Las Vegas) Raiders, famously said, "You can't teach speed." Lucky for you, Al Davis was wrong. Speed *can* be taught. And it *can* be learned. In fact, not only can speed be learned—along with strength, agility, balance, and proprioception—but it's essential that any athlete looking to achieve his or her maximum potential do just that.

WHAT'S THE SPEEDRUNNER SYSTEM?

THE SPEEDRUNNER SYSTEM is a 4-week, 12-session program designed to improve your athletic performance. There are also modified schedules for athletes focused solely on speed (e.g., team-sports athletes already enrolled in agility and strength-training programs), endurance athletes looking for a once-a-week combination speed- and injury-prevention workout, and fitness enthusiasts who'd like additional, stand-alone sessions beyond the initial program.

SpeedRunner creates positive training adaptations by teaching your nervous system to better control your muscles and connective tissue (e.g., your bones and tendons). It targets three physical skills that are a requirement for every sport.

SPEED	STRENGTH	AGILITY
Your ability to accelerate from your first step through maximum velocity	Your ability to generate force using your nervous system and muscles	Your ability to change direction rapidly

Of course, it all begins with speed. Speed is a dividing line in sports, like height requirements for amusement park rides. Once you have speed—the ability to move from point A to point B faster than others on the field, court, or track—you're already, literally, a step ahead of the competition. Add strength and agility, and you have a skill set that's prized in every sport.

The SpeedRunner system grew out of my own five-decade involvement in sports. I was a multisport athlete growing up, but my turning point in workout philosophy dates back 35 years to my time in Eugene, Oregon (America's track mecca), where I was training as a middle-distance runner. A friend of mine who ran with Nike's elite Athletics West program would meet me once a week under the bleachers at Hayward Field—rain beating down on the track, our breath like fog in the frigid temps, both of us bundled in sweats—and teach me the technique drills he'd learned with the club. We'd skip, bound, march, and do the Ovett Drill (a variation of Quick Feet named after one of the world's best milers), alternating reps of each drill with a sprint, for roughly two hours. The workout was designed to create nervous system adaptations that result in a more efficient stride. And, voilà, the next day my stride would be smoother and my pace faster.

A few years later, I was training at Brignole Fitness Club in Pasadena, California, which was owned by 1986 weight-class champion in the AAU Mr. America and Mr. Universe competitions, Doug Brignole. One of my workout partners, John, a beefy offensive lineman for a local junior college, a monster who bench-pressed more than 500 pounds, took me aside and said, "Pete, Ohio State's offered me a scholarship, but only if I can drop three-tenths off my 40." He knew I was a high school track coach—and that my team had won the league championship due to the domination of my sprinters. "Can you help me?"

I designed a program to get John those three-tenths, one that included the Oregon drills and other exercises. In the end, John signed with a Southern California school. But my interest was piqued: Just how much could a program that targeted nervous system adaptations improve speed in non-track athletes?

Flash forward to the summer of 2015. I put the results of years of training, coaching, and research to the test, finalizing the SpeedRunner system and offering it to

Speed in Sports

Different sports use different metrics to define speed. The NFL Scouting Combine uses the 40-yard dash. FIFA utilizes the top speed reached during a match to rank its fastest athletes. In track & field, the Olympic 100-meter champion has traditionally been declared the world's fastest human. To see how a few well-known athletes from a few different sports compare, let's break down each sport's unique metrics into miles per hour (mph) and kilometers per hour (kph):

Football	40-YARD DASH TIME	NFL COMBINE
Bo Jackson	4.12* sec.	19.86 mph or 31.96 kph
Chris Johnson	4.24 sec.	19.29 mph or 31.04 kph
Deion Sanders	4.27 sec.	19.17 mph or 30.88 kph

* Jackson's time might not have been run at the NFL combine, and there is conjecture that his time might also have been inaccurately recorded. (Jackson himself, during a 2016 ESPN His & Hers interview, claimed to have run 4.13.)

Tennis	TOP SPEED WHEN SPRINTING 3+ YARDS DURING A MATCH
Novak Djokovic	22.38 mph or 36.02 kph
Andy Murray	21.67 mph or 34.87 kph
Roger Federer	16.17 mph or 26.03 kph
Simona Halep	14.31 mph or 23.04 kph
Maria Sharapova	12.81 mph or 20.61 kph
Serena Williams	12.75 mph or 20.52 kph

Soccer	TOP SPEED RECORDED DURING A MATCH
Gareth Bale	22.93 mph or 36.9 kph
Cristiano Ronaldo	20.88 mph or 33.6 kph
Lionel Messi	20.19 mph or 32.5 kph

Track & Field	100-METER DASH TIME	VARIOUS MEETS
Usain Bolt	9.58 sec.	23.35 mph or 37.58 kph
Carl Lewis	9.86 sec.	22.69 mph or 36.51 kph
Jesse Owens	10.20 sec.	21.93 mph or 35.29 kph
Florence Griffith Joyner	10.49 sec.	21.33 mph or 34.32 kph
Shelly-Ann Fraser-Pryce	10.73 sec.	20.85 mph or 33.55 kph
Evelyn Ashford	10.76 sec.	20.79 mph or 33.46 kph

>>

Baseball	HOME PLATE TO FIRST BASE TIME	FASTEST RECORDED TIME
Mickey Mantle	3.10** sec.	19.80 mph or 31.87 kph
Billy Hamilton	3.52 sec.	17.44 mph or 28.07 kph
Mike Trout	3.53 sec.	17.39 mph or 27.99 kph

** Mantle's mark was hand-timed in the early 1950s, and there is no film or official timing data available to validate the mark—even so, Mantle was universally considered to be the fastest man in baseball during this period.

While it's impossible to reliably compare a football player's 40-yard dash and a soccer athlete's top speed (i.e., the former represents acceleration and the latter maximum velocity), it's safe to say that all these athletes are fast. If you're curious, the top speed ever recorded during an athletic event belongs to Usain Bolt, who clocked 27.8 mph (44.72 kph) from 60 to 80 meters during the 100-meter final at the 2009 Berlin World Championships in Athletics.

30 local high school student athletes. On Day One, all athletes were evaluated using four metrics tests:

1/ 40-yard dash   2/ 20-yard shuttle   3/ 3-cone drill   4/ Standing broad jump

The first test measured speed. The next two measured agility. The fourth measured explosive horizontal and vertical force. After four weeks of training, the student-athletes were tested again. Of those who had completed the entire program, 40-yard dash times improved by an average of 9 percent, with only one athlete failing to improve and all others lowering their times by at least three-tenths of a second. In the other tests, improvement varied between 10 and 15 percent.

There's nothing magical about the SpeedRunner program. Your nervous system controls your muscles. When you improve your nervous system's control of your muscles, while strengthening those muscles and their associated connective tissue (the tendons that connect each muscle to bone), you get faster, stronger, and quicker.

❯❯ NEUROMUSCULAR

Jointly using your nervous system and muscles; nervous system control of your muscles to create speed, strength, and agility

LET'S TALK THE SPEEDRUNNER SYSTEM

THE SPEEDRUNNER SYSTEM teaches your nervous system to use your muscles more effectively and efficiently. In Chapter 5, we'll cover this neuromuscular process in depth. For now, it's important that you have a general understanding of how this process works to produce movement.

As an athlete, you produce movement like this: Your nervous system sends signals to your muscles, your muscles contract, and then those muscles pull on tendons that connect to bones, altering the angle of your joints (e.g., bending a knee, straightening a hip, or flexing an elbow). Your nervous system doesn't control each muscle in isolation. Instead, it activates groups of muscles—what's called a "motor module"—in a specific sequence. It's those sequences that control movement. When you exercise using specific movements to generate speed, strength, and agility, your nervous system becomes more effective and efficient at recruiting the best motor module sequences to perform those skills. You get faster, stronger, and quicker.

How fast can these new nervous system activation patterns emerge? A 2016 study had subjects attempt a gait (similar to marching) with which they had no experience. By monitoring the subjects, the researchers were able to detect significant changes in neuromuscular activation "within the first few strides of attempting the new gait pattern" (Ranganathan et al. 2016). This indicates that the subjects' nervous systems began adapting immediately, experimenting with more efficient ways to perform the new gait.

A 1998 study defines this "initial, within-session improvement phase" as "fast learning" (Karni et al.). That's followed by a period during which your nervous system consolidates what it has learned, which might take several hours. After that, "slow learning" occurs, a process that might last days, weeks, months, or years—"consisting of delayed, incremental gains in performance emerging after continued practice."

SpeedRunner utilizes your nervous system's ability to adapt as both a "fast" and "slow" learner. By the end of your first session, you'll already be developing nervous

>> **SPEED**

The rate at which you self-propel over the ground; your ability to accelerate
(i.e., increase speed) or maintain a high maximum velocity (i.e., top-end speed);
a performance goal of being faster than your competition

system adaptations that will improve your performance. By the start of your second session, those adaptations will be absorbed. (Anyone who's practiced shooting free throws, skipping rope, balancing a barbell during weightlifting, or performing other athletic skills can vouch for the improvement that occurs between sessions.) By the end of your four-week program, the accumulation of *all* your adaptations will be hard-wired into your neuromuscular system. Best of all, those adaptations will stick with you as you segue into practice for your primary sport. Or, if you prefer, you can continue training the SpeedRunner way with weekly stand-alone sessions designed to maintain your fitness and continue your neuromuscular development.

One last point: Consistency and repetition are big parts of the SpeedRunner system. Consistency—building on previous fitness gains before they're lost by not skipping workouts—is like walking up the down escalator. Climb faster than the steps descend, and you reach the top. Take too long a break, and the escalator carries you right back to where you started. Repetition is how initial adaptations become hardwired. By performing specific movements over and over, your neuromuscular system becomes better at controlling them. This doesn't mean doing the same exercises every session. SpeedRunner includes variety, but it's a variety that reinforces gains you've already made, hardwires neuromuscular activation patterns, and builds incrementally toward a faster, stronger, and quicker you.

Let's Talk SpeedRunner Training

The SpeedRunner system Core schedule breaks your training into four categories of exercises and drills—acceleration, maximum velocity, strength, and agility—and then makes each category a focus for at least one of your three sessions per week:

Session 1	Session 2	Session 3
ACCELERATION & STRENGTH	AGILITY (including balance and proprioception) & STRENGTH	MAXIMUM VELOCITY

Note that all sessions include training for all categories. Acceleration relies on enormous leg strength to provide the push that fuels your first steps. Agility is, by definition, a form of acceleration (as you'll discover in Chapter 6). Maximum velocity is largely dependent on your ability to generate eccentric strength (see "Eccentric Running Wins the Race," page 15)—not to mention that the only way to achieve maximum

Peak Height Velocity: They grow up so fast!

Peak Height Velocity (PHV) is a fancy term for the period in life when adolescents experience their fastest growth—you know, when they sprout like weeds. Puberty. Girls tend to experience PHV earlier than boys, beginning at around age 11. According to the Centers for Disease Control and Prevention (CDC), girls gain an average of 2 to 4½ inches (5.4 to 9 cm) in height per year during this period. Boys don't reach PHV until about age 13, but they grow more once they get there, averaging 2½ to 5 inches (5.8 to 13.1 cm) per year. For coaches, parents, and young athletes, this raises a question: How will PHV affect training?

PHV is driven by an increased release of growth-related hormones, which are chemical messengers within your body that govern all aspects of biological function. Hormones are secreted by your endocrine system, then enter your bloodstream and travel to muscles, tendons, bones, organs, glands, and other tissues. Once there, they exert a multitude of effects. Many performance-enhancing drugs (PEDs), banned by almost every professional and amateur sports organization in the world, are either hormones or synthetic versions of hormones. During PHV, both boys and girls experience a huge increase in human growth hormone (HGH), which builds muscles, strengthens bones, and determines height. Boys also get an enormous bump in testosterone, a muscle builder and the mother of all steroid PEDs, with girls seeing smaller increases.

This combination of surging HGH and testosterone makes PHV an ideal time to introduce new types of training. A 2014 study found that 12 sessions of resisted sled towing produced big improvements in speed, leg stiffness, and force production in young athletes who were mid- or post-PHV, while pre-PHV study participants saw no improvement. Multiple studies concur that PHV is the time when athletes begin to see the benefits of resistance training, whether that's weight-sled work or pumping iron in the gym. The same studies advise restricting pre-PHV athletes to nervous-system-oriented training, like plyometrics and unresisted sprinting.

There's no denying that PHV opens the door for big fitness gains. Because of this, it's been called a window of opportunity, although there's no solid evidence that similar gains can't be generated post-PHV.

As a parent, coach, or athlete, you should keep in mind that any changes in a strength and conditioning program should be based on biological age (i.e., once PHV has begun) and not on chronological age. After all, some boys don't hit puberty until age 14 or 15. It's about the volume of muscle-building hormones in the bloodstream, not the candles on the birthday cake.

velocity is to accelerate. And general strength training stabilizes your body during all athletic movements, as well as being your number one defense against sports injuries.

SPEEDRUNNER SYSTEM FOCUS

The SpeedRunner system's primary focus is speed and agility. For strength, Speed-Runner offers training to stabilize your body during sprints and change-of-direction movements (i.e., agility), promote injury prevention, and improve whole-body strength (e.g., legs, core, and upper body) to the level required for successful team-sports participation. Athletes from some sports—such as football, rugby, and the weight events in track & field—might need to schedule additional sessions in the gym to increase their bulk muscle strength.

SPEEDRUNNER TRAINING SESSIONS

The SpeedRunner training sessions are designed to be performed at local schools, parks, or anywhere that has enough open space to let you run unobstructed for 30 to 40 yards. Two types of exercises and drills are offered:

> **Props:** These exercise and drills require equipment, such as weight sleds and medballs. They're geared toward athletes who are part of athletic programs or have access to props (e.g., through a gym or purchase).

> **No-props:** These exercises and drills require no props. All you need is a pair of shoes, and now and then a few stand-in props—for instance, paper plates in place of cones. Substitutes for props are offered in Appendix B, "Props, No-Prop Options, and Prop Swaps" (page 259). Additionally, all "props" exercises have a "no-props" alternative.

YARDS VERSUS METERS

All measurements are given in yards (unless I am referring specifically to the track, in which case I will use meters, or to scientific studies that relied upon meters for the purpose of measurement). If you are used to meters, don't let this confuse you. A meter and a yard are interchangeable in setting up your training:

$$1 \text{ meter} = 1.09361 \text{ yards}$$

For untimed exercises and drills, you can use meters simply by switching the recommended yards to an equal number of meters. For example: 15 to 20 yards = 15 to 20 meters.

Each session should last between 20 and 60 minutes, depending on the length of your warm-up, your recovery time between the exercises, and the specific exercises scheduled for that session. You should always feel free to add additional recovery between exercises.

SpeedRunner Book

The SpeedRunner book introduces you to the SpeedRunner system. It lays out the foundation for training, explains each targeted skill in depth, and details the kinds of training that most benefit each skill. Here's a peek at the chapters to come.

▸ **Chapter 2:** We break down the gait cycle (i.e., your running stride), and examine how SpeedRunner training addresses each phase of that cycle.
▸ **Chapter 3:** We look at acceleration, the most important phase of speed for most athletes.
▸ **Chapter 4:** We tackle maximum velocity, your top-end speed.
▸ **Chapter 5:** This is the strength chapter—we discuss how the nervous system and muscles work together to produce force.
▸ **Chapter 6:** Along with agility, we discuss balance and proprioception, which make agility possible.
▸ **Chapter 7:** This chapter offers a quick breakdown of your energy systems (how each fuels speed, strength, and agility), and methods for increasing speed endurance.
▸ **Chapter 8:** We talk recovery—most athletes fail to understand that you don't improve while you're training, you improve while you're recovering.
▸ **Chapter 9:** Here you'll find photo instruction for all exercises and drills included in the SpeedRunner schedules.
▸ **Chapter 10:** All of the schedules are found in this chapter.

SpeedRunner Metrics Testing

Metrics testing is how SpeedRunner tracks your progress. You don't have to test, but if you'd like to monitor your improvement from pre- to post-training, then the following metrics tests, performed in the order listed, will do the trick.

> **40-Yard Dash:** Tests acceleration (40 yards is also far enough for most team-sports athletes to reach maximum velocity)
> **Standing Broad Jump:** Measures explosive horizontal and vertical force
> **20-Yard Shuttle:** Measures lateral agility
> **3-Cone Drill:** Measures horizontal and lateral agility

Take at least a 3-minute break between each test (that's how long it takes to restock the energy system you'll be using). Breaks as long as 10 minutes are okay. Feel free to add tests of your own (e.g., vertical jump) but always begin with the four tests listed above. Also, limit additions to one or two tests, as nervous system fatigue will negatively impact your performance with more than 4 to 6 tests. Full instructions for each metrics test are included in Chapter 9.

SpeedRunner System Results

You should begin to improve during your very first SpeedRunner session, although significant and long-term improvement will require the full four weeks. Keep in mind that although your nervous system begins to adapt within seconds of starting an exercise or drill, it will take your muscles and connective tissue longer. They'll require at least 48 hours to fully repair post-workout, and it will take weeks before incremental gains result in noticeable adaptations.

CHAPTER 1 FINAL WORD

The SpeedRunner system is a science-based, experience-tested, 21st-century training program designed to improve any athlete's performance and fitness—no matter the sport. Equally beneficial to youth and adults, SpeedRunner targets adaptations in the nervous system to build speed, strength, agility, balance, proprioception, and explosive power.

2

SPEED: HUMAN LOCOMOTION

Human locomotion doesn't come easy.

Sure, it *seems* simple. You're sitting on the couch, binge-watching the latest Netflix series on TV. Suddenly you want a snack. So you hit "pause" on the remote, rise to your feet, and walk to the kitchen. Once there, you grab some dried fruit, unbuttered popcorn, or seaweed crackers—or doughnuts or Ho Hos or Cheez-Its. And then you walk back to the couch, sit down, and press "play." Nothing to it.

Except, of course, that there was a *lot* to it.

During that one simple journey, you orchestrated an unfathomably complex alliance of nervous system, muscles, joints, balance, proprioception, energy production, and more.

❯❯ HUMAN LOCOMOTION

Using your limbs to propel your center of mass (i.e., a point representing the average location of all the mass that makes up your body) across a given distance; crawling, walking, or running

Let's face it: Your capacity to self-propel is a marvel. Your body has been constructed from the inert elements of our planet's surface crust, yet you can move at will. You can travel from point A to point B. You can even *sprint* that distance. This latter capacity has evolved over the past four million years, beginning with our pre-*Homo* ancestor *Australopithecus*, who climbed down from the trees to stroll the African savannah at speeds of about 1 yard per second, a little slower than modern humans walk. After countless adaptations and mechanical improvements—better tendons, bigger butts, more sweat, less body hair—we humans now emerge from the womb as mostly pre-assembled human locomotion machines, with all the parts required to walk, run, or endure an ultramarathon. Just add food and water.

Yet while this capacity to self-propel is inherited, your mastery of locomotion is not. That's learned. And learned the hard way. Consider your own journey. At a few months old, using the process of trial and error, you managed to roll over for the first time. Next, you learned to crawl. And then, to walk. Barely a year old, you could toddle for short stretches. It took practice. It took patience. It took perseverance. And it took an amazing amount of pain tolerance, with research showing that infants average 17 falls per hour. *Ouch*, right? As you approached year two, you learned to run—engendering a few more spills, when your toddler-flawed forward lean put your feet behind your center of mass (a science-y term for the midpoint of your body's mass, which in a perfect sphere would be the exact center), necessitating a quick acceleration forward as you attempted to right your ship, with gravity eventually prevailing and you pitching face-first to the floor.

Years passed, and all that practice paid off. You graduated to racing siblings or friends through the house, chasing soccer balls on the playground, and suffering through the obligatory timed mile in eighth-grade PE. For those readers who've graduated the youth leagues, there were sports in high school, intramurals in college, and pick-up basketball, adult soccer leagues, and weekend 5Ks in perpetuity. Locomotion was fun. It was efficient. And you were as fast as you could get using the process of trial and error.

Satisfied, you declared your mastery of human locomotion complete. Only it wasn't. There was one level left to achieve: speed.

Eccentric Running Wins the Race

When you think about muscle contractions, you probably think about flexed biceps, fitness models flashing six-pack abs, or your quads and glutes aching after you carry a couch up a flight of stairs. That type of contraction—where a muscle flexes and shortens—is just one type of contraction. There are three:

▸ **Concentric contraction:** Your muscle shortens during contraction, producing force as it overcomes any resistance [e.g., your biceps flex when you curl dumbbells, creating big round mounds where your biceps pack together on your arms].

▸ **Eccentric contraction:** Your muscle lengthens [stretches] during contraction, producing force without being able to match or overcome an external force [e.g., you only get those dumbbells halfway up, then the weight starts to win—you eccentrically contract your biceps as your arms drop, your elbows straighten, and your biceps lengthen].

▸ **Isometric contraction:** Your muscle's length doesn't change during contraction, producing force without altering the angle of adjacent joints [e.g., the stationary plank position during core training].

During running, your leg muscles generate both concentric and eccentric contractions, usually with the latter preceding the former. And that's important. You see, when an eccentric contraction immediately precedes a concentric contraction in a muscle, that creates what's called a "stretch-shortening cycle," which increases the force of the concentric contraction. To illustrate how this works, think of how you'd approach a vertical jump test [i.e., you start from a standing position, then leap as high as you can]. You wouldn't squat, hold the position for a few seconds, and then jump. Instead, you'd quickly squat, then immediately reverse direction, springing into the air. This is known as a counter-movement jump. Dropping into the squat contracts your quadriceps, glutes, hamstrings, and calves eccentrically [they lengthen at the same time they're contracting—if they didn't contract, you'd drop straight onto the ground]. Springing right back up flexes them concentrically. Counter-movement jumps add more than 10 percent to the height of your vertical leap [and swinging your arms adds another 10 percent].

The same stretch-shortening phenomenon is at work when you run.

>>

16

▸ **Hamstrings:** Your hamstrings contract eccentrically as you lower your foot toward the ground, then quickly switch to concentric contraction right before footstrike, helping to pull your leg back and, once on the ground, move your center of mass forward.

▸ **Quadriceps and calves:** When you land, your quadriceps and calf muscles contract eccentrically, lengthening as your knee and ankle bend to absorb your landing, then quickly shift to concentric contractions to push you back into the air.

▸ **Hip flexors:** As your leg stretches behind you, foot on the ground, your hip flexors (the muscles that bring your knees toward your chest) resist the stretch with an eccentric contraction, then quickly shift to a powerful concentric contraction that drives your knee forward and into the next stride.

▸ **Glutes:** Your glutes contract eccentrically as your knee rises ahead of you, slowing that rise, then quickly shift to a concentric contraction that brings your thigh back down toward the ground.

In sum, you use eccentric contractions to set up the concentric contractions that power running. Consequently, stronger, more intense eccentric contractions lead to stronger, more intense concentric contractions, which in turn lead to faster running.

WHAT'S SPEED?

SPEED IS THE ACT OF ACCELERATING QUICKLY to top-end velocity and then maintaining it. Simple, right? Just like crawling, walking, and running, right? Sorry, wrong. Because unlike other forms of bipedal human locomotion, you can't master speed through trial and error. You won't get there by toddling along and avoiding falls. You can only achieve speed with specialized training that targets every aspect of human locomotion: your nervous system, your muscles, your connective tissue (e.g., tendons), your energy systems, and the gait they produce.

If all there was to running fast was natural ability honed by friendly competition on schoolyard fields, athletes like Usain Bolt, world record-holder and three-time Olympic champion at 100 and 200 meters, wouldn't have trained 21 hours per week in the gym and on the track. Jerry Rice, the NFL's all-time greatest receiver, with 197 receiving touchdowns and 1,549 career catches, wouldn't have spent his off-seasons on The Hill in Redwoods City, California's Edgewood Park, mixing long runs and hill sprints to create speed and speed endurance. And Lionel Messi, one of the greatest footballers of all time, with five Ballon d'Or awards and three European Golden Shoes, wouldn't rely upon workouts jam-packed with jump squats, plyometrics, short sprints, and other exercises to build acceleration, top-end speed, and multi-directional agility.

With a commitment to proper training, your speed can be improved, too. "[Your ability to run fast] is influenced by a multitude of factors," write Aditi Majumdar and Robert Robergs, the latter one of the world's leading exercise scientists, in a 2011 article on speed, "including starting strategy, stride length, stride frequency, physiological demands, biomechanics, neural influences, muscle composition, [and] anthropometrics." That's a lot of factors. And still it barely scratches the surface of what we'll explore in this book. Again, this is a good thing. The more factors we can legitimately identify, the more opportunity there is to improve those factors through training.

This is the first of three chapters on speed. We'll focus on acceleration in Chapter 3 and maximum velocity (i.e., top-end speed) in Chapter 4, but we'll begin our look at speed by breaking down the most fundamental unit of running, your gait cycle. The running gait cycle begins when you land on one foot and ends when you land on that same foot again. The gait cycle is also called a stride. However, since runners use *stride* interchangeably to refer to an actual stride (your gait cycle) and a step (which begins when you land on one foot and ends when you land on the opposite foot), it's less confusing, in this one instance, to use the science-y term. So gait cycle it is.

We'll look at both the series of movements that make up the gait cycle itself and the processes which drive those movements. In order, we'll tackle the following:

▹ **The spring-mass model:** the classic theory of how your running gait cycle operates, in which stride is viewed as analogous to a pogo stick
▹ **Active versus passive running:** comparing running gait to a human slingshot
▹ **The stretch-shortening cycle, stretch reflex, and elastic recoil:** three ways in which your body's passive mechanisms drive the gait cycle
▹ **Phases of the running gait cycle:** the movements your body goes through during a single turn of the gait cycle

Do you really need to know all this stuff to get faster? No, you don't. You can proceed straight to the SpeedRunner training schedules in Chapter 10 and reap the benefits of the system. But understanding how your body works to produce speed

18

(and strength, agility, and energy) serves two purposes. One, it will give you confidence that your workouts are targeting the correct muscles and mechanisms. Two, it will help you mold training sessions of your own, if the book's schedules don't perfectly match your needs. Rest assured that we'll keep these chapters simple. This isn't a science textbook, and there won't be end-of-chapter quizzes. Yes, we'll use some science-y terms, but you don't have to memorize them—use the index to find an explanation where they first appear.

LET'S TALK SPEED AND HUMAN LOCOMOTION

BEFORE WE TALK ABOUT THE MECHANISMS that drive the gait cycle—or even about the phases of the gait cycle itself—I need to be honest with you: There isn't universal agreement about what occurs during each running stride. A lot of the disagreement stems from the fact that the gait cycle changes as your running gait changes. For example, the gait cycle is different during acceleration and steady-pace running. And it's different when you're jogging or sprinting. A researcher monitoring your gait cycle during jogging would record a huge contribution to propulsion (pushing off the ground with your back leg) from your calves and quadriceps. A researcher monitoring you while you sprinted would credit propulsion to your hamstrings and glutes. Both would be right. The point is that the gait cycle—the muscles, mechanisms, and strategies involved—isn't consistent over all paces. That's a big reason why this book has a chapter each for acceleration and maximum velocity—because they aren't the same thing.

But there are a lot of things about the gait cycle that are consistent and upon which there is agreement. Whenever there's disagreement on topics covered in this book, I'll try to cite sources and studies for the currently prevailing theories. The good news is that while theories change, the underlying training that works stays pretty much the same—we just come up with better reasons for why it works.

The Spring-Mass Model

The spring-mass model theorizes that when you run, your legs work like a pogo stick. A real pogo stick has an internal spring that compresses each time the pogo stick lands on the ground, then subsequently decompresses, releasing all the energy stored during compression and launching the pogo stick—and joyful rider—back into the air. If you've ever ridden a pogo stick, you know that it's a combination of spring and rider effort (pushing down with your legs during compression, pulling up on the handlebars during decompression) that creates the best bounce possible.

19

You employ the same pogo-stick principle when you run. Your body compresses as you land on your foot—in this case storing energy, called elastic energy, in your muscles and tendons—and then, as you begin to accelerate upward again, your body combines a release of this stored energy with active muscle contraction to send you sailing into the air.

The main springs are your tendons—in particular, the Achilles tendon. Unlike the springs in a pogo stick, your tendons stretch rather than compress upon landing. Still, the result is the same: Stored energy is released to aid locomotion.

The spring-mass model holds for most people whether they're jogging or sprinting, with the exception of elite sprinters, who veer from the model as their speeds climb above 7 meters per second. While most runners generate maximum force about 50 percent of the way through contact time (i.e., the length of time your foot is on the ground), equivalent to the pogo stick at its most compressed, world-class sprinters reach maximum force in half that time. We'll discuss this in Chapter 4. For now, understand that 99 percent of runners abide by the spring-mass model.

Active Versus Passive Running

Jay Dicharry, a leading expert on running mechanics, has characterized the running gait cycle as a "human slingshot." From this perspective, a passive mechanism like elastic energy storage-and-release is seen as a strategy to be wielded by athletes. "Hold the slingshot," writes Dicharry in *Anatomy for Runners*, "pull back on the elastic band, aim, release and—*whap!* Rock hits target."

Whether it's your Achilles tendon absorbing energy and then—*whoosh!*—releasing that energy as you push off your foot and launch into the air, or your leg being stretched back on the ground before—*zing!*—being rocketed forward by the stretch-shortening cycle and stretch reflex, these are passive mechanisms that occur outside your conscious control. Let's look at a simple distinction between active and passive mechanisms.

- **Active mechanisms:** muscular contractions, such as flexing your biceps, that require conscious control.
- **Passive mechanisms:** actions, such as elastic recoil, that occur outside your conscious control.

Active mechanisms are easy to recognize. For instance, you stand at the start line, someone yells "Go!" and you push off one leg with all the power you can muster. Passive mechanisms are more complicated, especially since they tend to overlap. But understanding how they contribute to running (and therefore speed) is fundamental to designing a training program. Let's look at three passive mechanisms that we'll revisit frequently in this book.

ELASTIC RECOIL

When one leg lands during running, your tendons, muscles, and ligaments stretch. As they do, they absorb what's called elastic energy. Think of Dicharry's slingshot. Stretching your tendons—especially your Achilles tendon—is like pulling back the slingshot. Once your foot passes beneath your body (placing it behind your center of mass), you release that stored energy, which combines with the force generated by your muscles to propel your body both up and forward. Best of all, this elastic recoil is free. The energy (think gravity) that causes your tendons to stretch is transformed into elastic energy. How much energy? In their 1998 review, Novacheck et al. report that an average-sized man running 6 minutes per mile stores 35 percent of the energy required for each stride in his Achilles tendon, another 17 percent in his arch, and more still in his quadriceps and patellar (knee cap) tendons. Added together, more than half the energy required for each stride is provided by elastic energy.

STRETCH REFLEX

Tiny stretch receptors called muscle spindles are located within your muscles, positioned parallel to your muscle fibers. These spindles sense changes in the length of your muscle fibers. When your muscles stretch beyond their desired length during exercise, these spindles increase the volume of their messaging to your spinal cord, and your nervous system responds by ordering the stretched muscle to contract, thereby protecting it from overstretching and damage. The stretch reflex transpires incredibly fast, in a mere 1 to 2 milliseconds. The reflex also inhibits muscles that oppose the new contraction—in other words, if a stretch reflex causes your quadriceps (front thigh muscles) to contract, it *also* instructs your hamstrings (back thigh muscles) to relax. The result is a more effective contraction. A classic example of the stretch reflex is the knee-jerk response. A physician uses a tiny hammer to tap the patellar tendon beneath your knee, which stretches the quadriceps above the knee and triggers a stretch reflex—the quadriceps contracts, and your lower leg jumps. While running, stretch reflexes contribute to locomotion almost every time a muscle is stretched.

STRETCH-SHORTENING CYCLE

When an eccentric contraction immediately precedes a concentric contraction in the same muscle, the result is a stretch-shortening cycle that increases the force of the concentric contraction (see "Eccentric Running Wins the Race," page 15, for an explanation of eccentric and concentric contractions). For example, when you land during running, your quadriceps lengthen (stretch) even as they contract (i.e., they contract eccentrically). If they didn't contract, stabilizing your knee, you'd crash to the ground. As your leg moves beneath your body, these same quadriceps muscles switch to a concentric contraction, shortening as they straighten your knee in anticipation of propelling your body back into the air. This stretch-shortening cycle increases the force your quadriceps can contribute to propulsion.

Mike Parkinson, a PT and sprint coach, suggests that athletes mistakenly assume that all their muscles fire all the time while they run. Instead, muscles flash on and off, like fireworks in the sky, generating big, short-lived contractions through both active and passive mechanisms—like those detailed above—to produce the fast, effective, and efficient rotation of our limbs known as the gait cycle.

Phases of the Running Gait Cycle

Your running gait cycle begins as soon as one foot touches the ground, and it includes all the movements of your lower body until that same foot touches down again. Since your legs mirror each other like spokes on opposite sides of a wheel, we'll follow a single leg through the gait cycle. Some runners display minor differences between legs, but those differences don't affect the basic mechanics we're outlining here.

We'll split the gait cycle into two phases: stance and swing. During stance, your foot is on the ground. During swing, it's off the ground. We'll further break down stance and swing into sub-phases. Different researchers, coaches, and athletes use slightly different terminology for these sub-phases, but everyone's addressing the same movements.

INITIAL CONTACT

Stance phase begins with initial contact. Initial contact begins the instant your foot touches the ground. Your footstrike occurs slightly ahead of your center of mass (imagine a point slightly below and behind your belly button—that's the approximate location of your center of mass during upright running). With initial contact, your body begins the process of braking (slowing down) and energy absorption. If your foot lands too far in front of your body, which happens when you overstride, you'll brake too much. If your foot lands directly under your hips, you'll sacrifice the elastic energy absorption that accompanies braking. At initial contact, your lower leg should be at a 90-degree angle to the ground. At slower paces, between 80 and 85 percent of runners land heel first. Speedsters, on the other hand, favor a mid-to-forefoot landing.

BRAKING

An instant after initial contact, your muscles, tendons, and other connective tissues absorb a ground reaction force (GRF). In accordance with Newton's third law of motion—"For every action there is an equal and opposite reaction"—this GRF is the ground's reaction to the force you exert upon it by landing. Consider it pushback. During normal running, the GRF can equal two to three times your body weight. For sprinting, that number can double. At slower paces, your knee bends during landing about 20 to 25 degrees. Top speedsters, on the other hand, might appear to experience no knee bend at all. This is due to *leg stiffness*, a concept we'll discuss in Chapter 4. As your knee and ankle bend, your calves and quadriceps contract eccentrically. Your Achilles tendon stretches, absorbing elastic energy. Your glutes and hamstrings stay busy extending your hip—for our purposes, think of "extending" as "straightening," which in this case means that the angle where your front thigh meets your pelvis straightens as your thigh moves backward.

MIDSTANCE

As your foot moves beneath your hips, the GRF reaches its peak, meaning that the force you're exerting on the ground also reaches its peak. Some runners mistakenly believe that peak GRF occurs at initial contact. It doesn't. At slower paces, your foot flattens on

>> **STANCE PHASE**
The part of each stride when your foot is on the ground (20 to 40% of the gait cycle)

Phases of Running

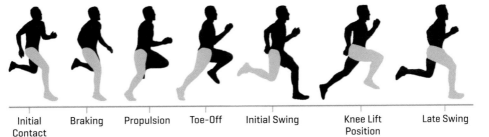

| Initial Contact | Braking | Propulsion | Toe-Off | Initial Swing | Knee Lift Position | Late Swing |

the ground by midstance, known as *foot flat*, while your knee flexion reaches approximately 45 degrees. At top speeds, your heel might never touch the ground, and the bend at your knee might mirror initial contact. Your center of mass reaches its lowest point (i.e., closest distance to the ground). If you were a plane, you'd have successfully landed. Of course, just like that, it's time to take off again.

PROPULSION

As your foot moves behind your hips, you apply propulsive force to the ground (once your foot is behind your center of mass, you're no longer braking). You combine elastic recoil from your Achilles tendon, arch, and patellar tendon (up to 95 percent of stored energy is released) with concentric contractions of your calves, quadriceps, and hamstrings to trigger a triple extension—the joints at your ankle, knee, and hip all straighten. Note that top speedsters will leave their knee slightly bent. Your hip flexors, the muscles that lift your thighs and knees, work eccentrically as your leg stretches behind your hips.

TOE-OFF

This is the moment your foot leaves the ground. For slower runners, toe-off occurs about 40 percent of the way through the gait cycle. For elite speedsters, it can happen as early as 22 percent into the cycle. Toe-off is the time when you'll optimize your flight path. It's like throwing a baseball. If you throw too high, the ball won't go far. If you throw too low, gravity will drag the ball straight into the turf. Exercise scientist, author, and coach Steve Magness advises watching the horizon as you push off. "If it stays flat, you are too horizontal. If it bounces a lot, you are too vertical." Find an effective middle ground. Go for what speedsters call *lift*, without bouncing like a bunny rabbit.

INITIAL SWING

Swing phase begins the instant your foot leaves the ground. A strong combination of stretch-shortening cycle and stretch reflex, triggered just before toe-off, causes your hip flexors to contract, creating a slingshot effect that pulls your thigh forward. Simultaneously, your lower leg, with your knee acting as a hinge, sails upward. At top speeds, your heel will nearly kick your butt (glutes)—a motion you'll mimic in the Butt Kicks drill (page 170) for maximum velocity training.

MIDSWING

As your knee passes beneath your hips, you retain the knee-tuck position from initial swing—about 90 degrees for distance runners and up to 130 degrees for sprinters, who tuck their lower leg closer to their thigh. This knee-tuck position serves a purpose: It makes it easier to swing your leg forward. Try an experiment with your arm. Extend one arm out from your shoulder, then swing it back and forth. Next, bend your elbow so that your hand is near your shoulder, then swing your arm back and forth again. Did your arm move more quickly with the second method? It's the same thing with your leg. With a good bend at your knee, you can bring your leg forward faster.

KNEE LIFT POSITION

As your thigh rockets ahead of your body, your hip flexors begin to throttle back, like booster rockets shutting down after a spaceship has cleared Earth's gravitational pull. Your glutes contract eccentrically to further slow thigh movement. Knee lift position occurs when your knee reaches its highest point in front of your body.

LATE SWING

It's time for your leg to descend. The combination of a stretch-shortening cycle and stretch reflex triggers a strong concentric contraction from your glutes, which are joined by your hamstrings in driving your thigh downward and extending (straightening) your hip. This downward force snaps your lower leg forward at the knee—a motion that's arrested by your hamstrings, which work eccentrically to maintain

>> **SWING PHASE**
The part of each stride when your foot is off the ground (from toe-off through initial contact)

some bend in the knee (otherwise, you'd end up executing a goose step). The eccentric load on your hamstrings reaches 6 to 10 times your body weight (see "Hammy Time," page 61, for the price your hamstrings pay for their role during late swing). And your quadriceps, calves, and other leg muscles spring into action, tensing as they prepare to absorb the landing GRF. As sprint coach Charlie Francis has pointed out, the key to being a top speedster is your ability to tolerate the shock of landing. Your hamstrings align your lower leg for a 90-degree landing, your hip continues to extend, your foot dorsiflexes (i.e., the top of your foot lifts toward your shin) . . . and this is where we started, at initial contact.

AERIAL TIME (FLOAT PHASE)

Aerial time refers to the two periods of swing phase—one immediately after toe-off and one preceding initial contact (with each referred to as a *float phase*)—when both your feet are off the ground. Your movement during aerial time is largely determined by passive mechanisms. Your hip flexors, which drive your knee forward during the float phase that immediately follows toe-off, are fueled by the stretch-shortening cycle and stretch reflex that preceded toe-off. You can't consciously improve that hip flexor contraction—you can only weaken it. Ditto for the hip extension that occurs during terminal swing, which relies on similar passive mechanisms (we'll explore these more in Chapter 4). Bottom line: During aerial time, heed a saying that's popular with pilots when your plane reaches cruising altitude: "Sit back and enjoy your flight."

CHAPTER 2 FINAL WORD

In their 1995 study, Wiemann and Tidow write that "the end stage of the motor evolution seems to be the synchronous and two-legged bounding behavior of the kangaroo, the one-legged alternating running behavior, without pelvis rotation, of ostriches, and the sprinting behavior of *Homo sapiens*, with rotation of the pelvis and contralateral arm swing." So you've already made the top three, species-wise, for locomotion simply by virtue of your swinging hips and arms. As you've seen in this chapter, however, there's a lot more to running gait than that. A smart athlete will view each phase and sub-phase of the gait cycle as an opportunity—an opportunity to identify the involved muscles and mechanisms, to focus on training that will improve both, and to become the speedster that trial and error, by itself, can't deliver.

25

3

SPEED: ACCELERATION

Acceleration is the most prized running skill in sports. And it's the phase of speed that every athlete utilizes.

"Only in track & field's 100- and 200-meters is top-speed running a key factor," says exercise scientist and sprint biomechanics expert, J. B. Morin, in a 2015 interview. "In all other sports—soccer, football, rugby, etcetera—much shorter distances represent most of the demands of the game, and very rarely do players actually reach their individual top speed."

If you compete in team sports, you know what Morin is talking about. Studies show that decisive sprints in team sports last less than 20 yards—and often less than 10 yards. A 2016 study found that half of all sprints in soccer last less than 10 yards, which is a good thing since the average player performed 150 to 250 of these 2- to 3-second accelerations per match. A 2012 study determined that in baseball, a batter's chance of

>> **ACCELERATION**

Your capacity to increase speed; the ability to gain speed within a short time; the rate at which you change velocity (speed in a given direction)

Acceleration by the Numbers

The acceleration phase lasts until the runner can no longer increase his or her speed, at which point the runner transitions into the maximum velocity phase. There are notable differences in how untrained runners, average speedsters (team-sports athletes or runners with some sprint training), and top speedsters (athletes with sub-elite or elite sprint training) handle the acceleration phase. Let's take a quick look at some comparisons by the numbers.*

Length of acceleration phase

Youth or untrained runner	10–30 yards
Average speedster	30–40 yards
Top speedster	50–75 yards

Number of steps required to achieve at least 50% of maximum velocity

Average speedster	3–4 steps
Top speedster	2 steps

Distance required to achieve 90% of maximum stride rate (cadence)

Top speedster	2 steps

Steps required to reach maximum power (power = force × velocity)

Top speedster	6–7 steps

Top speedsters' horizontal force production compared to average speedsters

First step	+25%
Average for all steps	+10%

Top speedsters' vertical force production compared to average speedsters

Average for all steps	-2%

>>

Number of strides required to achieve maximum velocity

Average speedster	10–14 strides
Top speedster	22–30 strides
Usain Bolt	30–32 strides

*All numbers based on statistics found in *The Mechanics of Sprinting and Hurdling* [Mann and Murphy], "Sprint Mechanics in World-Class Athletes: A New Insight into the Limits of Human Locomotion" [Rabita et al.], a 2015 interview with J.B. Morin, and other sources.

The numbers show that the best speedsters apply greater horizontal force more quickly from the very first step of acceleration, and then they continue to accelerate for a longer period of time than less talented, trained, and fit athletes.

beating a throw to first base was most affected by his acceleration from home plate to the foul line—a distance of just 45 feet (15 yards). And in the NFL, home of America's speediest team-sports athletes, research found that a player's 10-yard sprint time was almost perfectly correlated to his 40-yard performance. In other words, an NFL player who could burn a fast 10 yards was good to go for 40—which is what really counts in a league in which less than 1 percent of plays go 40 yards or more.

Mike Boyle, a strength and conditioning coach whose resume includes the 2013 World Series Champion Boston Red Sox, the NHL's Boston Bruins, and numerous Olympic team-sports champions, sums it up best in his book, *New Functional Training for Sports*: "Sport is about acceleration, not [top-end] speed."

WHAT'S ACCELERATION?

ACCELERATION AT ITS MOST BASIC is the act of increasing your running speed. From a standing start (or blocks), you explode into action. If you're already running, you pick up the pace. Acceleration continues until you can no longer increase your speed, at which point you achieve maximum velocity (top-end speed).

Acceleration seems simple enough. You want to go faster, so you run harder. In reality, acceleration requires a different gait cycle than steady-pace running, an emphasis on powerful concentric contractions (at least at the start), and, most importantly, enough newly generated force to overcome inertia.

In the last chapter, we mentioned Newton's third law of motion: "For every action there is an equal and opposite reaction." To understand inertia, we turn to Newton's first law of motion: "A body continues in a *state of rest* or uniform velocity unless acted upon by an external force." For acceleration, the state of rest equates to a motionless start—that is, a standing, 3-point, or 4-point start. *Uniform velocity* is the steady pace you're running before you accelerate. Both represent inertia. Neither can change until you generate enough force to overcome them—to accelerate.

So what's acceleration? It means applying enough force to the ground to increase your speed.

Most of what we know about acceleration comes from sprinters, sprint coaches, and studies on sprinters. That doesn't mean the knowledge isn't relevant to speedsters outside the sport of track & field. The acceleration mechanics practiced by the world's top sprinters are, by and large, the same mechanics you'll use (or should use) in your sport. Sure, you'll run with a slightly lower center of mass, less knee lift, and less knee flexion (bending) when agility is required, but anytime you explode for a 5- to 20-yard burst, you'll want to be acceleration-trained according to the same gold standard that produces elite sprinters.

In this chapter, we'll cover the basic ingredients of acceleration:

▸ **Horizontal force:** the key to forward acceleration
▸ **Braking force:** deceleration while your foot is in front of your center of mass
▸ **Concentric leg strength:** the muscle-factor key to first-steps acceleration
▸ **Phases of acceleration:** different phases require different mechanics and specific training
▸ **Acceleration training:** the nuts and bolts for building improved acceleration

Acceleration lasts between one to five seconds in team-sports contests. No matter how many hours you put into every other skill required for your sport, success in your sport comes down to those seconds. Or, more accurately, it comes down to the tenths-of-a-second advantage you'll need over your competition.

❯❯ INERTIA (IN RUNNING)

Your body's resistance to a change in motion, whether you're trying to begin moving from a motionless start or to increase your speed while on the fly

LET'S TALK ACCELERATION

THE FIRST THING YOU NEED TO KNOW about acceleration is that it involves a big push.

Imagine that your car just broke down, but you can see an auto repair shop just down the road. Inertia dictates that unless you apply force to the car, it will remain at rest. So you decide to push. Your friend will steer. You lean into the car, hands on the trunk, feet planted behind you, and you concentrically contract your leg muscles as hard as you can. In other words, you push. Your reward for that effort is that the car rolls forward.

The first steps of acceleration are like that. Acceleration requires a huge amount of force in the forward—or horizontal—direction. In other words, a push.

Horizontal Force

The next thing you need to know about acceleration is that your ability to produce this push in the forward direction is determined by three external forces: the ground reaction force, gravity, and wind resistance (with the latter two factors working against you). Since there's not much you can do about gravity or wind resistance, let's focus on ground reaction force, or GRF.

Recall that GRF is the force the ground exerts on you in response to the force you exert upon it. What we didn't discuss is that the GRF exerts its force in three different directions: vertical, lateral, and horizontal. While running, vertical force gets you back into the air. Lateral force helps you sidestep defenders—when discussing running speed, we can ignore lateral force. And horizontal force propels you forward.

Given that acceleration requires a huge push forward, it seems obvious that horizontal force should be the key factor during this phase of speed. And recent studies bear this out.

"In the blocks," says Morin, "elite sprinters produce much more—about 25 percent more—horizontal force and power than less skilled sprinters. When averaging data from all the steps of the [acceleration phase], we observe that faster sprinters produce 10 percent higher horizontal forces." In a 2016 study, Morin is blunter: "Faster athletes were those who pushed the most in the horizontal direction."

In contrast, vertical force plays only a small role during acceleration. In fact, a groundbreaking 2005 study by Hunter et al. concluded that you only need enough vertical force to get off the ground and then stay in the air long enough to reposition your legs. More force than that was a waste of time and energy.

To summarize: During acceleration, you need enough vertical (upward) force to stay in the air while you switch legs, and the rest of your effort should go into generating horizontal (forward) force. Later in this chapter, we'll discuss training that will help you do just that.

Before we leave horizontal force, there's one other thing you should know: When you reach maximum velocity, everything flips. Vertical force becomes king, and horizontal force is a blip on the GRF radar.

Braking Force

In Chapter 2, we broke down stance phase (when your foot is on the ground) into a braking phase and a propulsion phase. The braking phase occurs from initial contact (when your foot first touches the ground) until midstance. You "brake" because your foot is in front of your center of mass—the ground reaction force pushes against you, attempting to move you in the opposite direction of the one you're facing, so you slow down. Once your foot passes beneath your body, the GRF switches direction. Now, it pushes you from behind, driving you forward.

When you subtract the amount of braking force (plus air resistance) from the amount of propulsion force, both of which are horizontal forces, you get the net horizontal force.

If that net horizontal force favors propulsion, you accelerate. If it's a wash, you maintain pace. If it favors braking (and air resistance), you slow down.

For your first step from a motionless start, braking accounts for only a fraction of the horizontal force. Consequently, you explode forward. But by step three, braking's percentage of horizontal force begins to grow. This happens for two reasons:

> **Stride length:** Your stride length increases with each step. Your first two steps land completely behind your center of mass, so there is negligible braking. At step three, your foot lands in front of your center of mass, and braking begins. With each step, you land a little farther in front of your center of mass, lengthening the braking phase—hence, allowing more braking force to develop. At maximum velocity, you'll devote about 50 percent of stance phase to braking (even top speedsters brake for 40 percent of stance).

Contact time: With each step, you spend less time on the ground—that is, stance phase shortens. Less time on the ground leaves you less time to create propulsion force.

The result of all this is that by the time you reach maximum velocity, the braking force (plus air resistance) and propulsion force are equal. The net force is zero. Acceleration ends.

Some form gurus suggest reducing braking forces by landing directly under your hips (your center of mass). Don't do that. Contact time (the time your foot spends on the ground) is already getting shorter as you accelerate. Shorten it more, and your muscles won't have time to develop their share of the force needed to propel you back into the air. Also, braking facilitates the storage of elastic energy, which, as you recall, provides half the energy you need for your stride. Finally, there's this: Hunter et al. found that the ability to generate greater propulsion force accounted for 57 percent of the difference between faster and slower runners, while an ability to reduce braking force was credited with a 7 percent effect. So sure, don't brake more than you have to, but never forget that acceleration is about generating a big push.

Concentric Leg Strength

In Chapter 2's examination of the gait cycle, we focused on the role eccentric contractions play in driving passive mechanisms like the stretch-shortening cycle. From a motionless start, however, acceleration is all about the strength of concentric contractions—muscle contractions in which the muscle shortens, like when you flex your biceps.

When you accelerate from a motionless start, you can't take full advantage of passive mechanisms like the stretch-shortening cycle. Unlike a countermovement jump for vertical height, in which you squat quickly (and eccentrically) before reversing direction to spring into the air, a motionless start requires that you compress the spring in your start position and then hold it—thereby losing stored elastic energy and negating any benefits of stretch shortening and stretch reflex. Instead, you rely on the ability of your quads, glutes, hamstrings, hip flexors, and calves, among other muscles, to produce powerful concentric contractions.

One 2015 study broke down the main components of initial acceleration and concluded that "the ability to produce a great concentric force/power [is of] primary importance" at the start of acceleration. You start from a crouched position and then drive forward explosively, utilizing a forward lean for your first steps (good sprinters use about a 45-degree angle coming out of the blocks). Your hip extensors (glutes and hamstrings) contract forcefully to move your body forward over your stance foot. Strong concentric contractions from your quadriceps and calves join those of your hip extensors to create a powerful triple extension of hip, knee, and ankle at toe-off, propelling you forward.

Legendary exercise scientist and sprint expert Ralph Mann, PhD, estimates that a top speedster will generate over half of his or her maximum velocity by the end of step two in acceleration, using these powerful, concentric contractions. Think about that: *two steps*. Two small steps in terms of distance covered, two giant steps toward your top-end speed.

Phases of Acceleration

As you've probably already gathered, acceleration isn't one single, unvarying phase. Instead, from your first steps to the final phase before maximum velocity, acceleration involves changes in posture, mechanics, and force production. Let's break it into three phases and look at it more closely.

FIRST STEPS

The first two to three steps of acceleration rely on powerful concentric contractions. From a 3-point or 4-point stance, your first two steps will fall behind your center of mass. From any motionless start, your ultimate goal is to reach one-half your maximum velocity by step two and 90 percent of your maximum stride rate (cadence) by step three. You'll lean forward, push hard, and minimize the time between steps.

TRANSITION PHASE (5 TO 20 YARDS)

Your stride lengthens, reaching about 80 percent of maximum length by 20 yards. Your body transitions to a more upright posture. Eccentric contractions resume their importance during the gait cycle, with the stretch-shortening cycle for your hamstrings critical to continued acceleration. With each step, the amount of horizontal force you can produce declines, and athletes who can continue to exert larger amounts of horizontal force start to pull away from the competition.

FINAL PHASE

As your production of horizontal force begins to reach an equilibrium (the point where braking force plus air resistance cancels out propulsion force), your rate of acceleration

>> **HORIZONTAL GROUND REACTION FORCE**

The horizontal part of the ground reaction force; a force that slows you during braking and accelerates you during propulsion; your ability to orient the GRF horizontally is the top predictor of acceleration performance

35

slows. At the same time, you must continue producing enough vertical force to get off the ground. Since your contact time (the time your foot is on the ground) progressively shortens as you accelerate, you have less time to produce horizontal and vertical force. At this stage, vertical force gets priority, and horizontal force decreases as a percentage of total force. To better utilize the GRF, speedsters employ leg stiffness (we'll talk more about this in Chapter 4)—stiffer knees and ankles are more efficient at absorbing and releasing energy. In a 2012 interview, Morin explains the value of leg stiffness by equating its opposite—running with more flexible hips, knees, and ankles—to having a flat tire. No matter how powerful your car's engine, you can't go very fast on flat tires. Likewise, you can't utilize muscle contractions and the GRF unless you have stiff legs. Finally, you reach the point where you can't produce enough propulsion to overcome braking, and acceleration ends.

LET'S TALK ACCELERATION TRAINING

DID SOMEONE SAY "PUSHING?" That's right, *we* did, over and over in this chapter. So it shouldn't come as a surprise that acceleration training will involve strengthening the muscles responsible for that push. You also want to perform exercises and drills that improve your horizontal force production through all phases of acceleration.

Training for Your First Steps

Acceleration training begins with strengthening your first few steps. Whether you begin from a motionless start or on the fly, the first few steps can determine the success of an athletic move during a game or practice. If you're using a motionless start, you'll need to practice the mechanics required to go from zero to sprinting. If you're accelerating on the fly, you'll still need to generate extra force for that first uptick in speed.

TRIAL AND ERROR

Okay, so I said proper speed training couldn't be learned through trial and error. And yet here we are, using trial and error to learn the mechanics of proper first-steps acceleration. The difference is that you'll specifically create situations that force you to execute proper mechanics—that is, these aren't exercises that occur regularly during most people's days. Training begins with the Push-Up & Sprint (page 132), in which you start from the push-up position, then scramble to your feet and launch into a sprint. Too often, we overanalyze the step-by-step components of exercise. By starting from the push-up position, you're forced to experiment with angles, muscle contractions, balance, and other processes that occur too quickly for conscious control. By repeating the exercise, you intuitively select those actions that create the most efficient movement. The Jump & Sprint (page 128) and Medball Push & Sprint (page 131) further develop your intuitive first-steps mechanics.

WEIGHT SLED PUSH

Boyle writes that if he "could do only one exercise, it might be a sled push... A weighted sled teaches strong athletes how to produce the type of force that moves them forward." In the Weight Sled Push (page 135), you can load your sled with as much weight as you want. Then you can push the sled at the same angle you'll use for the first steps of a standing, 3-point, or 4-point start. You'll train your muscles in the same way you'll use them during competition.

HILL SPRINTS OR STADIUM STEPS

If you don't have a weight sled at your disposal, then Hill Sprints and Stadium Steps (page 130) are a terrific stand-in. Exercise scientist, writer, and speed coach Patrick Beith explains on his website, "Hill work is perfect for acceleration development, as it puts the athlete in proper acceleration mechanics." The ground rises up to meet you at the same angle you'd utilize for forward lean during acceleration. Plus, by fighting gravity, you put your legs through a strength workout. If you don't have a steep hill, then use the stadium steps at a local school. "Running every other step on the bleachers mimics acceleration mechanics similar to short hill work," says Beith.

WEIGHTED JUMPS

On the surface, weighted jumps—for instance, Jump Squats (page 174) with a weight vest or dumbbells—are a vertical force exercise. After all, you jump up and down. Nevertheless, numerous studies have found strong correlations between weighted jumps

Acceleration Training—Useful Exercises for Phases of Acceleration

Different exercises target different phases of acceleration. The shaded line indicates which segments of a 40-yard acceleration are most affected by the specified training (e.g., sled pushing benefits the first 5 yards).

EXERCISE	0–5 yd.	6–10 yd.	11–20 yd.	21–30 yd.	31–40 yd.
Heavy Resistance Training	■				
Weight Sled—Pushing	■				
Weighted Jumps	■	■	■		
3-Point Starts & Initial Acceleration Drills	■	■	■		
Weight Sled—Marching	■	■	■	■	
Hill Sprints	■	■	■	■	■
Weight Sled—Pulling		■	■	■	■
Resistance Harness Sprinting		■	■	■	■
Countermovement Jumps			■	■	■
Non-resisted Sprinting			■	■	■
Plyometrics			■	■	■

and your ability to produce force during first-steps acceleration from a crouched position. "Contrary to popular belief," writes Mann, explaining this correlation, "the start involves the production of balanced levels of horizontal and vertical forces." That's because you're not just moving your center of mass forward at the start, you're also raising it as you rise from a crouched to an upright posture.

PROPER STARTS

Some team-sports athletes utilize a 3-point stance (page 125). And all SpeedRunner athletes who participate in metrics testing will want to learn it, the better to blaze your 40-yard dashes. You can also practice a 4-point stance by including the 3-Bounce & Run (page 124) exercise.

HEAVY RESISTANCE TRAINING

The SpeedRunner system doesn't include heavy resistance training (e.g., free weight squats, deadlifts, and cleans). That doesn't mean heavy resistance training doesn't work. Studies show a definite correlation between first-steps acceleration and resistance work that stresses lower body muscles with near-maximum loads. SpeedRunner provides the same initial strength gains with exercises and drills that target nervous system adaptations. For long-term muscle strengthening—and especially for athletes in sports like football—supplemental workouts at a local gym might be warranted.

Training for Acceleration's Transition and Final Phases

During the remainder of acceleration, you incrementally transition to an upright posture, lengthening your stride, shortening your contact time, and maintaining as much forward-directed horizontal force as possible. Resistance work and neuromuscular training are your top priorities.

RESISTED RUNNING

Resisted running helps develop your horizontal force-generating capacity.

Three of SpeedRunner's resisted running exercises require props, either a resistance harness and tether or a weight sled. If you don't have access to those props, visit Appendix B (page 259), or substitute extra sets of countermovement jumps, plyometrics, and 90-percent strides. You do resisted running exercises for one main reason: They improve your ability to generate horizontal force. Exercises in the program include Weight Sled Run (page 138), Resisted Run (page 129), Hill Sprints and Stadium Steps (page 130), and Weight Sled Marching (page 136).

COUNTERMOVEMENT JUMPS

Countermovement jumps work the stretch-shortening cycle, stretch reflexes, and elastic recoil. A 2006 study examined the relationship between the countermovement jump and the first 10 meters of a sprint. It found that the "explosive ability" of quadriceps, glute, and hamstring contractions during a countermovement jump could "predict 10 m sprint performance." While we used weighted jump squats for first-steps training, Jump Squats using only body weight is a good exercise for transition and final phase acceleration. To add more horizontal orientation to your countermovement jumps, try the Standing 5-Jump (page 134).

PLYOMETRICS

Plyometric exercises provide excellent training for the transition and final phase of acceleration, but they're even more useful for maximum velocity, so we'll cover them in Chapter 4.

BOUNDING

Although technically a technique drill (and regularly performed along with the other technique drills you'll find in Chapter 4), Bounding (page 127) has such a strong horizontal component that it needs to be included here. A 1994 study of sprinting and bounding concluded that bounding "seems to be a specific strength exercise for sprinters... because of its short contact time, great propulsive horizontal force, and consequently high power."

SPRINTING

Unresisted sprinting is an effective exercise for improving the second half of acceleration. You need to run at 90 percent or more of your top-end speed, although faster than 90 percent is not necessarily better. Sure, you'll need to blow out your pipes now and then. But 90 percent of top speed will provide you with the same neuromuscular benefits as faster training—with less nervous system fatigue. You'll recover more quickly, so you'll be ready to train again sooner.

CHAPTER 3 FINAL WORD

You've been introduced to a lot of concepts in this chapter. Sometimes, this much data can be overwhelming. But the main takeaway is pretty simple: Train to push harder, more effectively, and more efficiently. That's it. And just because we listed a gazillion exercises in the training section doesn't mean you must start by doing all of them. And you won't—not if you follow the schedules in Chapter 10. Morin compares initial speed training to having a full tube of toothpaste: "When the toothpaste is full (low skill level), no matter how you press the tube (no matter how you train) you'll get some toothpaste (performance improvements). So any kind of force training might result in sprint performance gains." That's where we are. You won't have to do much at first to improve. Later, as the tube empties and your skill level begins to max out, Morin warns that you'll "have to press the tube with very specific and well-designed gestures" to continue improving. But that's a wonderful problem to have. Imagine being so fast and powerful during acceleration that you'll need an Olympic-level coach to eke out a bit more. For now, focus on pushing past your competition by pushing harder during bursts of acceleration.

4

SPEED: MAXIMUM VELOCITY

Faster than a speeding bullet. More powerful than a locomotive…

No, you're not Superman, but you'll need Superman's lightning-quick feet and enormous capacity for generating force if you're going to improve your maximum velocity. For acceleration, your primary objective is to push—harder and more effectively than you've ever pushed before. For maximum velocity, you have an equally simple objective: to hit the ground as hard and fast as you can.

"When sprinting, your goal should be to put as much force into the ground as possible to move forward as quickly as possible," writes Andrew Sacks in a 2013 website post. Sacks has trained athletes of all ages and skill levels, from nine-year-olds to college stars to major league baseball players on rosters for the Cubs, White Sox, Twins, Orioles, and Diamondbacks.

Hit the ground hard and fast. It's that simple.

>> **MAXIMUM VELOCITY**

Top-end speed; the highest possible sprint speed you can achieve, usually short-lived

But is it necessary?

In the last chapter, we identified acceleration as the key phase of speed for most athletes, and we acknowledged that team sports generally don't require sprints that extend beyond this acceleration phase. So why train for a type of speed you'll rarely, if ever, use on the field or court? Because when you train to be faster at longer sprints, you'll also get faster at shorter sprints. Maximum velocity training accomplishes this by increasing both the distance you're able to accelerate and the horizontal force you can produce with each step. The result: You end up faster, from your first step to your last. As sprint researcher and coach Ken Clark explains in a 2017 interview, "There is no better way to train the nervous system than high-speed running because it [requires] the highest rate of force application." So to train your nervous system for all phases of speed, maximum velocity running offers the biggest return. Besides, as Clark reminds team-sports athletes: "When big plays happen, they're often based on whose top speed is fastest." It's up to you to determine which side of those "big plays" you'd like to be on.

WHAT'S MAXIMUM VELOCITY?

MAXIMUM VELOCITY IS TOP-END SPEED. It's that moment when you can no longer accelerate. Until that moment, the positive (forward) horizontal force you've been generating has been larger than the negative (opposing) force—the negative force is a combination of braking force and drag (air resistance). At maximum velocity, these positive and negative forces equal out. You can't get any faster. But neither are the negative forces enough—yet—to slow you down.

At top-end speed, you've still got inertia on your side—a body in motion will stay in motion. All you need to do is produce the minimum horizontal force required to offset braking and drag, while also producing the necessary vertical force (think up and down) to get you off the ground at toe-off. As your contact time (the time your foot is on the ground) for each step gets shorter, you must produce force quicker. That requires a shift to an upright posture and a change in gait cycle mechanics, which we'll address shortly.

One other thing: Maximum velocity ends almost as soon as it begins. While it takes an Olympic sprinter 50 to 60 meters (i.e., 55 to 65 yards) to reach maximum velocity, he or she can only maintain that speed for 10 to 30 meters (i.e., 10 to 33 yards). You may last 10 to 20 yards. After that, deceleration begins. It doesn't seem fair. All that work

Maximum Velocity by the Numbers

Maximum velocity begins where acceleration ends. The period during which you can sustain maximum velocity is short-lived, lasting about 10 to 30 yards, but a look at how average runners (untrained or endurance-trained runners), average speedsters (team-sports athletes or runners with some sprint training), and top speedsters (athletes with sub-elite or elite sprint training) cover those yards explains the gulf that lies between them.

Advantages held by top speedsters over average runners

Stride length	+70%
Stride rate (cadence)	+20%
Ground reaction force	+25%

Percentage of gait cycle at which toe-off occurs

Average runner	40%
Average speedster	25–35%
Top speedster	20–22%

Duration of maximum velocity phase

Average speedster	10–20 yards
Top speedster	10–35 yards

Characteristics of a top speedster*

Stride length (men)	2.75–2.9 yards
Stride rate (men)	4–5 steps per second
Stride length (women)	2.2–2.5 yards
Stride rate (women)	4–5 steps per second

Minimum ground contact (stance) time

Average runner	300 milliseconds
Average speedster	120–135 milliseconds
Top speedster	90–100 milliseconds
Fastest speedster in the world	80 milliseconds

>>

Minimum swing time

Average runner	345 milliseconds
Fastest speedster in the world	320 milliseconds

Minimum aerial (float) time—same for all runners

Acceleration phase	40–50 milliseconds
Maximum velocity phase	125–130 milliseconds

Energy cost from drag (air resistance)

Marathoner	2%
Miler	4%
Sprinter at maximum velocity	8%

Force generated at maximum velocity

Average speedster	3–4 × body weight
Top speedster	4–5 × body weight
Usain Bolt	1,000+ pounds

All numbers are averages and some have been rounded; figures are based on statistics found in *The Mechanics of Sprinting and Hurdling* (Mann and Murphy); "Sprint Mechanics in World-Class Athletes, A New Insight into the Limits of Human Locomotion" (Rabita et al.); "Usain Bolt: Case Study in Science of Sprinting" (Hart); various studies conducted by Peter Weyand et al.; and other sources.

* For these figures, a "stride" equals one stance phase plus the following aerial phase (i.e., one step).

What do all these numbers mean? Basically this: The best speedsters apply greater vertical force more quickly, leading to shorter contact times and faster stride rates, even as they also achieve longer stride lengths. Regardless of top-end speed, all runners have the same minimum aerial time. That means it's what you do on the ground that counts.

for 10 to 20 yards of top-end speed? But look at it this way: You get 30 to 40 yards of high-quality acceleration before reaching maximum velocity, so altogether you'll blast 40 to 60 yards *before* the slow-down kicks in.

Speaking of Olympic sprinters, only Usain Bolt has come close to sustaining maximum velocity through 100 meters. For everyone else, it's a matter of limiting deceleration. When you see a sprinter burst into the lead over the final meters of a 100, he or she hasn't picked up the pace. Instead, the other sprinters are fading faster.

Researchers aren't sure why top-end speed is so short-lived. Acceleration expert Morin speculates that "you're getting neuromuscular fatigue which lowers your vertical and propulsive forces." He also suggests your feet and ankles get tired—that's the "flat tire" analogy from Chapter 3. Of course, "fatigue" is a tricky concept; no one's sure what causes it. The Central Governor theory suggests that your brain shuts down muscle fibers when energy supply is low, body heat is high, etc. But the specific anaerobic system that provides most of the energy for sprints is good for 10 to 12 seconds of explosive burn—surely long enough to carry an Olympic sprinter past 60 to 80 meters (and average speedsters past 50 to 60). And you don't overheat in 10 to 15 seconds. Another theory suggests it's the process of creating the energy itself that leads to fatigue. Whatever the reason, fatigue happens. And when it does, your speedometer moves backward.

We'll discuss energy systems more in Chapter 7 and fatigue in Chapter 8. For now, let's stick to the components of maximum velocity.

- **Vertical force:** In maximum velocity, it's all about hitting the ground hard.
- **Knee lift position:** What goes up (higher) must come down (harder).
- **Hip extension:** The engine for maximum velocity resides in the hip extensor muscles.
- **Contact time:** Less is more.
- **Leg stiffness:** You want stiffness from your toes to your shoulders.
- **Stride length versus stride rate:** The right mix makes you a faster sprinter.
- **Asymmetrical gait:** For elite speedsters, the spring-mass model goes out the window.
- **Stability:** Speedsters don't wobble.

While you may never reach maximum velocity per se in your sport, the trickle-down effect of maximum velocity training will improve your acceleration and overall running efficiency. You'll get faster. You'll get fitter. And you'll be on the high-fiving end of those big plays.

⟫ VERTICAL GROUND REACTION FORCE

The vertical (think up and down) component of the ground reaction force (GRF); the vertical force the ground exerts on you, equal to the vertical force you exert on it; if you stand still, the vertical force is equal to your body weight

LET'S TALK MAXIMUM VELOCITY

DURING ACCELERATION, your mission was to create propulsive horizontal force. You needed big, strong pushes to propel yourself to faster speeds. Now, at maximum velocity, your goal is to produce enough vertical force to stay in the air between steps, while also creating the modest amount of propulsive force required to maintain top-end speed. Easy, right?

"The ability of sprinters to apply ground forces of 4 to 5 times the body's weight in less than one-tenth of a second without losing their balance, while reversing direction of the center of mass, and with negligible fluctuations in horizontal velocity during each stance phase, requires both great skill and high-level musculoskeletal function," writes exercise scientist, coach, and masters (age 40+) sprinter Jimson Lee on his website, SpeedEndurance.com.

Okay, so maybe not so easy.

Step-by-Step Instructions for Hitting the Ground Hard and Fast

Hitting the ground hard and fast is the key to maximum velocity. But as simple as that objective sounds, Lee is right: The ability to generate competitive-level top-end speed is a remarkable skill. Your legs are whirling. Both your feet are off the ground more than they're on it. It's all you can do to maintain balance and run a straight line. How can you be expected to execute a hard, fast footstrike up to 4 to 5 times per second? The answer is that no one could—if you are expected to consciously stomp the ground each time your foot completes another circuit. Instead, that goal footstrike is the end result of an entire gait cycle, a sequence of active and passive actions that you'll teach your body during training and then set in motion when you're ready to sprint. To understand exactly how that process works, let's start at the end of a stride, as your foot hits the ground, and then work our way backward.

FOOTSTRIKE

A stride begins when your foot hits the ground. But during maximum velocity, a stride also ends there, as each turn of the gait cycle has a single purpose: to generate a hard, fast footstrike that will maintain top-end speed.

A 2000 study on the importance of vertical GRF to sprinting found that "speed is conferred predominantly by an enhanced ability to generate and transmit muscular force to the ground."

Coach Clark puts it in layman's terms, "We should be able to hear that pop on and off the ground. If [your foot] is mushing into the ground, that's not good."

At maximum velocity, horizontal force accounts for a measly 10 percent (or less) of total GRF, with lateral force a tenth of that. The rest is vertical force. In the short period of time available to generate GRF (about three-hundredths of a second for top speedsters, up to twice that long for you), you'll need to apply between 3 and 5 times your body weight to the ground—that is, if you want to get back into the air and maintain your velocity.

The 2000 study focused on sprinters whose top speeds ranged between 6 and 11 meters per second. It found that even small increases in vertical force produced huge increases in speed. Only 5 percent more vertical force netted an increase in top speed of 1 meter per second. If you project that out, you net 10 meters for 10 seconds. That 10-meter improvement is enough to turn a good high school sprinter into a national-class athlete.

That's a lot of bang for your vertical force buck.

But increased vertical force doesn't come from nowhere. To see how you generate a hard, fast impact force, let's rewind a fraction of second.

TERMINAL SWING

An instant before initial contact, your leg is extended almost to the ground. There's a slight bend at the knee, but your hamstrings are contracting eccentrically to prevent your lower leg from snapping completely forward. If your knee did straighten, your foot would land too far in front of you, creating an extended braking phase guaranteed to slow you down. At this instant, your leg is descending so quickly that your hamstrings endure a load 8 to 10 times your body weight to hold your knee in place. Just before footstrike, your hamstrings switch to concentric contraction, utilizing a stretch-shortening cycle to create a furious backward pawing action of your leg. This backward action hammers your foot into the ground—you hit the ground hard and fast. Of course, this result only occurs if your leg is, indeed, descending at breakneck speed. To see how this speed is generated, let's rewind again.

KNEE LIFT POSITION

Peter Weyand, one of the authors of the 2000 study on sprinting, said in an interview, "We found that the fastest athletes all do the same thing to apply the greatest forces needed to attain faster speeds." Weyand, one of the world's top experts on maximum velocity, added, "They cock the knee high before driving the foot into the ground."

It's the height you achieve during knee lift position (when your knee is at its highest point in front of your body) that determines how fast your leg descends. High knee lift accomplishes this in two ways:

1/ It increases the distance your foot will travel to the ground, giving your leg more time to accelerate.

2/ It triggers intense stretch-shortening cycles in your glutes and hamstrings, resulting in powerful concentric contractions that hurl your thigh toward the ground.

Of course, you don't accidentally achieve higher knee lift. It's the result of a passive action that occurs way back at toe-off.

TOE-OFF

You don't consciously hoist your knee high. Instead, you use Dicharry's slingshot concept to launch it forward from toe-off. As stance phase ends, your hip hyperextends so that your leg can trail behind your body. This backward movement of your leg stretches your hip flexors—the muscles responsible for bringing your thigh and knee forward. Just before toe-off, a fast, forceful hip hyperextension triggers an equally forceful stretch reflex in your hip flexors. This stretch reflex combines with a strong stretch-shortening cycle to drive your thigh forward, an action that lifts your knee in front of your body. Of course, the key to this hip flexor contraction is that fast, forceful hip extension. To see how that's generated, let's rewind one last time.

HIP EXTENSION—POWER

Long before your foot contacts the ground, your hip extensors (glutes and hamstrings) begin pulling your thigh back (remember, extending your hip means straightening the angle where your pelvis meets the front of your thigh). As your foot touches the ground, the extension continues. Your glutes—what sprinters call "the engine"—contract until mid-stance. At that point, your hip begins to hyperextend (your thigh angles backward as your foot moves behind your body), and your hamstrings become the prime movers.

The faster you run, the more your hip extensors become responsible for leg motion. A 2012 study found that hip extensor contribution doubled from 7 meters per second to 9 meters per second. A 2015 study credited glutes and hamstrings with the "predominant role as running speed increased and reached high [7-meters-per-second] to maximal sprint speeds."

When we're talking about "forceful" hip extension at maximum velocity, we're talking about the concentric contractions of your glutes and hamstrings.

HIP EXTENSION—SPEED

"At high running velocities," writes Morin on his website, "the only action leading to a backward push of the foot on the ground is violent hip extension."

It's not enough for your glutes and hamstrings to contract powerfully during stance phase. They must also contract *violently*, which requires a combination of power and quickness. How quick? Per step, top speedsters spend less than 0.1 second on the ground.

For comparison, when you're out on a jog, your contact time (the time you spend on the ground) is about 300 milliseconds, or three-tenths of a second. When you sprint at top speed, that probably drops to about 120 to 135 milliseconds. A top speedster does the same in 80 to 100 milliseconds. Think about that. Top speedsters are zipping from initial contact to toe-off, while executing a powerful hip extension that creates enough vertical force to get them back into the air, in about two-thirds the time it takes you to do the same.

Of course, there's a reason you spend longer on the ground than top speedsters. The reason is that you need that much time. In the 120 to 135 milliseconds it takes you to complete stance phase, your muscles are only capable of generating about 50 percent of their maximum force—which is just enough to get you back in the air and moving forward. At 80 to 100 milliseconds, you'd be lucky to create enough propulsion to get off the ground at all, let alone complete another stride.

So how do top speedsters do it?

They hit the ground hard. Even though top speedsters generate only 20 to 50 percent of their muscles' potential force during contact time, they strike the ground so hard that they're able to create their peak GRF in a fraction of the time it takes slower runners. They're already packing their bags for the next flight while the rest of us are waiting for the pilot to turn off the "fasten seatbelt" sign for the current one.

They maintain leg stiffness. When top speedsters strike the ground, their bodies don't fold at the joints.

"Think of bouncing a beach ball versus a super ball," writes Jay Hart, in an article on Usain Bolt. "The beach ball is soft and mushy and when bounced on the ground sits for a while.... Conversely, a super ball is hard and stiff and when bounced rebounds almost instantaneously—and at a much faster speed than that beach ball."

That's leg stiffness in a nutshell. Be a super ball. Not a beach ball.

"When it's time to go, we gotta make sure they are not mushing into the ground," says Clark, talking about leg stiffness in his athletes. "When we strike the ground, we are aggressively stopping that lower limb with a really stiff ground contact on the ball of the foot and staying stiff all the way up through the chain, whether it's ankle, knee, hip, torso, shoulders, etc.—whether that's acceleration or top speed." According to Clark, the principle is equally valid for Olympic sprinters and team-sports athletes.

If you watch world-class sprinters in full flight, one thing you won't see is bending at the ankle or knee when their feet strike the ground. With lightening quickness, they absorb and release forces, producing stretch-shortening cycles at hyperspeed. They're human super balls.

HIT THE GROUND HARD

Which brings us back to the beginning of this rewind—to the instant your foot hits the ground. Now that we've seen how this force was produced, let's run the film forward:

- You strike the ground hard on the ball of your foot.
- Leg stiffness restricts flexion (i.e., bending) at your ankle, knee, and hip, generating a large GRF quickly and facilitating more rapid stretch-shortening cycles and elastic recoil.
- A shortened ground contact period increases your rate of hip extension.
- A violent hip extension triggers an intense hip flexor stretch reflex.
- Your hip flexors catapult your thigh forward, leading to a high knee lift position.
- Powerful hip extensor contractions hurl your thigh toward the ground.
- The extra distance to the ground created by high knee lift position allows your leg to generate more speed.
- Greater speed results in a stronger stretch-shortening cycle for the hamstrings as your foot nears the ground.
- The speed of descent plus a last-instant concentric hamstring paw-back of the lower leg allows you to (drumroll please) hit the ground hard and fast.

And round and round it goes.

Stride Length Versus Stride Rate

We can't discuss top-end speed without touching on an age-old debate: What's the best way to increase speed? There are two options:

▸ Increase your stride rate (also called "stride frequency" and "cadence")
▸ Increase your stride length

The problem with this debate is that the two alternatives are not separate strategies. Both are achieved through one simple action: You hit the ground hard. Still, let's take a quick look at each component.

STRIDE RATE

When athletes talk "stride rate," they're really talking "step rate." To athletes, a "stride" occurs every time you take a step. They aren't concerned about gait cycle analysis or lingo. Distance runners measure stride rate in steps per minute (e.g., many shoot for a cadence of 180 steps per minute). Speedsters measure it in steps per second. Olympic sprinters can manage almost five steps per second—a little over two-tenths of a second for each step. You probably can't match an Olympic sprinter's stride rate. But here's something you can match. Top speedsters require a minimum of 125 to 130 milliseconds for each float phase (the time both feet are off the ground). And you? 125 to 130 milliseconds. That's right, you and Usain Bolt spend the same amount of time in the air. The difference in your stride rate and Bolt's is determined by your respective contact times. Bolt spends less time on the ground than you do. It takes him less time to develop the force necessary to get back into the air and maintain horizontal velocity. If you want to spend less time on the ground, too, you'll have to hit the ground harder.

STRIDE LENGTH

Again, when athletes talk "stride length," they really mean "step length." Your stride length, in athlete-speak, is the distance between the initial contact of one foot and the initial contact of the other. If you and another athlete take the same amount of time to run a stride (i.e., your stride rates are the same), but you travel farther with each stride, then you run faster. Of course, there's a big "but" there. The assumption is that you can maintain the same stride rate. In reality, it takes more time on the ground (for athletes of similar ability) to produce the force required for a longer stride—hence, longer strides lead to slower stride rates. A 2010 study comparing one-legged hopping

Usain Bolt Versus Bo Jackson

It's one of the long-running debates in American sports: Who'd win a race at 40 yards, the reigning Olympic 100-meter champion or the best players in the NFL, considered home to America's fastest team-sports athletes? Lucky for us, sprint coach and writer Carl Valle has come up with the answer. Using a velocity analysis, and adjusting for factors like running surface and timing equipment, Valle estimates that three-time Olympic Champion Usain Bolt, at his peak, ran the 40 in 3.96. In contrast, the NFL combine's official record for the 40-yard dash is 4.22, set by John Ross in 2017, with the unofficial record belonging to Bo Jackson, with his 4.12 in 1986. Keep in mind, too, that Bolt still had almost 70 yards left to run (i.e., 100 meters equals 109 yards) when he posted his time. So until NFL players can break the 4-second barrier, this race belongs to the Olympic champ.

to sprinting found that while hopping produced vertical forces that were 30 percent greater than those generated while sprinting—creating a whopper of a stride length—the sprinters kicked the hoppers' booties. That's because the sprinters ran two steps for every one hop. "Maximizing speed," the study concluded, "involves a trade-off between the magnitude of the ground forces applied and the step frequencies that can be attained." In general, top speedsters and almost-top speedsters generate similar stride lengths. They both hit the ground hard enough to produce the required vertical force—top speedsters just hit it a tiny bit faster.

Asymmetrical Gait

Asymmetrical gait applies only to the very best speedsters in the world. But it's worth taking a peek for the rest of us. The spring-mass model predicts that GRF will peak at mid-stance, forming a perfect upside-down "U" on a graph. But that model goes out the window for world-class sprinters. Elite sprinters hit the ground so hard and fast that some produce a GRF peak as early as 22 percent of the way through stance phase, compared with 45 to 50 percent for the rest of us. A chosen few exhibit two peaks, one at 20 percent and the second at roughly 50 percent. Those peaks are also larger than those of sub-elite speedsters. It's beyond the scope of this book to explore the mechanics or training required for such feats, but if you'd like to watch extraordinary footage of speed in action, there are great videos on the Southern Methodist University Speed Lab YouTube channel: www.youtube.com/user/LocomotorLabSMU.

Stability

Attaining top-end speed requires good posture and efficient whole-body movement. Toward that end, the following components play a role.

Core muscles: At top-end speed, your legs and arms move furiously. A strong core (muscles located in your back, abdomen, and pelvis) keeps you from spinning out of control. It supports your upright posture, keeps your lower back and pelvis properly angled, and controls every movement, from bending to twisting to knee lift.

Arms: Arms should swing to counterbalance your legs. The backward swing triggers a stretch reflex in your chest and shoulders, causing your arm to slingshot forward. Your hand should rise to about eye level. It's an old runner's tale that you should drive your arms hard when you're trying to run fast. Instead, working your arms only interrupts the stretch reflex, wastes the energy involved in flexing muscles, and slows you down.

Balance and proprioception: You can't run fast and straight if your balance and proprioception are off. We'll explore both in Chapter 6.

Exercises that address stability will be included in Chapter 5, "Strength."

>> **LEG STIFFNESS**
The ability to keep your legs from flexing (bending) at the knee, ankle, and hip during stance phase; the use of straighter limbs to avoid energy loss, to maximize elastic recoil, and to shorten contact time

LET'S TALK MAXIMUM VELOCITY TRAINING

SPEED PLAYS A HUGE ROLE in most team sports, but practice sessions for those sports rarely include training for speed. Instead, you train at sub-maximal levels, with no specific targeting of acceleration and maximum velocity skills. The long-term result is that you de-train your ability to produce speed. That's right: By practicing for your sport, you get slower. SpeedRunner reverses speed losses and improves maximum velocity by training you for vertical force production, violent hip extension, elastic recoil, and more efficient top-end running form.

Technique Drills

Technique drills isolate and exaggerate elements of your sprinting gait cycle. Top speedsters have used them for generations. But that doesn't mean they aren't without controversy. Magness writes on his blog, "Drills are not useful for improving mechanics because they do not replicate the running form biomechanically, neurally, or muscle recruitment wise."

In contrast, Dicharry has written that "individualized drills and neuromuscular activities... will train [runners] to use elastic recoil in gait." And a 2009 study concluded that a mix of running drills, agility exercises, and explosive starts led to "significant improvement" in the participants' neuromuscular control. But the main reason you should include SpeedRunner drills in your training is that the fastest men and women in the world include drills in theirs. When you perform your drills, keep in mind that the fast stride that follows each drill is essential to hardwiring the drills' benefits into your sprinting performance.

SKIPPING DRILLS

Both Skipping (page 164) and High Skipping (page 165) stimulate elastic recoil in your Achilles tendon and arch, with the latter drill also orienting the elastic recoil vertically, the better to develop vertical force.

HAMMER AND NAIL DRILLS

These drills develop knee lift, late-swing hip extension, leg stiffness, and elastic energy absorption. Flat-Footed Marching (page 166) elevates knee lift position through two nervous system adaptations: reduced inhibition (we'll cover this concept in the next chapter) and reduced sensitivity of the muscle spindles that trigger stretch reflexes.

High Knees (page 167) work the triple-combo of leg stiffness, elastic recoil, and elevated knee lift position. Bounding is an excellent drill for developing both vertical and horizontal force capacity, as well as knee lift and elastic recoil. It also strengthens your quadriceps and calves eccentrically, crucial for supporting your weight during initial contact and braking.

CONTACT TIME DRILLS

In their seminal 2010 study, Weyand et al. write that the upper limit on your maximum velocity potential is not determined "by the maximum forces the limbs can apply to the ground, but rather by how rapidly they can do so." It's about hitting the ground hard *and* fast. Quick Feet (page 168) taxes your nervous system with an ultra-quick foot shuffle. Quick Hops (page 169) includes a plyometric element, forcing you to employ rapid-fire stretch-shortening cycles and elastic recoil to power a series of short, low-to-the-ground hops.

BUTT KICKS

This is a great exercise to finish a set of drills. You strengthen muscles involved in early swing, plus you dynamically stretch your quadriceps—which also makes this a great warm-up exercise (page 170).

Vertical Force and Leg Stiffness

Hitting the ground hard and fast are not separate elements of sprinting. One leads to the other. Leg stiffness allows you to transform the speedy descent of your leg into an almost instantaneous large vertical force. An efficient stretch-shortening cycle quickly absorbs that force and then returns it, leading to a powerful and shortened contact time.

PLYOMETRICS

Plyometric exercises are also known as "jump training." You begin from an elevated height, drop to the ground, absorb the landing force, and then immediately spring into a vertical jump. It's a countermovement jump with an extra twist—an elevated start height. Plyometrics train your nervous system and muscles to absorb more force and to make the switch from eccentric to concentric contractions more efficiently. These exercises improve leg stiffness, elastic recoil, vertical force production, and the strength of the involved muscles. If you have access to plyo boxes, the Depth Jump (page 173) is the most effective plyometric exercise. Double-Leg Hops (page 180) and Single-Leg Hops (page 181) are the poor man's version of depth jumps.

REPEATED HOPPING

Coach Valle writes that "hopping on one leg repeatedly, jumping on two legs, or alternating between legs is helpful for many athletes who lack elastic power." The Triple Hop on 1 Leg (page 172) offers strong elastic recoil work, while also developing vertical and horizontal force production. Exercises like Ankle Poppers (page 178) and Weighted Ankle Poppers (page 179) train ankle stiffness and improve the endurance you'll need for maintaining that stiffness through extended sprints.

COUNTERMOVEMENT JUMPS

The Jump Squats exercise (both body weight and weighted, pages 174–175) is excellent training for vertical force production.

Hip Extension

Much of our training for hip extension was included in Chapter 3's acceleration training, and there's more to come in Chapter 5. For now, let's finish maximum velocity training with two exercises and one drill.

WALKING LUNGES

Walking Lunges (page 176) strengthen the muscles (e.g., quadriceps, hamstrings, and glutes) you'll use to generate top-end speed. You'll also target vertical force as your center of mass rises and falls with each lunge.

STRAIGHT-LEG BOUNDING

Straight-Leg Bounding (page 171) rehearses the hip extension you'll tap from knee lift position through initial contact. You'll use a strong glute-hamstring extension to drive your leg toward the ground, then an equally focused hip flexor action to return your leg to its start position. This is a great strengthening exercise for both hip extensors and hip flexors.

STRIDES (90%)

This is a carryover exercise from acceleration training. At 90 percent effort, you'll activate most of the same motor modules in the same sequences required for maximum velocity running. A 2011 study documented a 5 percent improvement in top-end speed through repeated-sprint training only. Numerous other studies have reported small to large improvements in power, speed, and endurance from repeated-sprint training. Valle sums it up best: "The most direct way to run faster is to simply sprint at different distances and at different speeds."

CHAPTER 4 FINAL WORD

Before picking up this book, you might have thought "speed" was simply pointing yourself in the right direction and letting fly. After three chapters on the topic, I'm betting you've changed your mind. If anything, Majumdar and Robergs' declaration that speed is "influenced by a multitude of factors" probably now seems an understatement. At the same time, you've also learned that—with a smart, methodical approach to training all the factors that affect acceleration and maximum velocity—you can and will get faster.

5

STRENGTH

There have been nine multiple-time champions of the World's Strongest Man competition. These men average six feet, three inches (190.5 cm) and 341 pounds (155 kg). To earn their place atop the podium, they bested their rivals in events like the Atlas Stones, which requires that five stones, ranging in weight from 220 to 400-plus pounds (100 to 180-plus kg), be heaved atop five incrementally taller platforms; the Car Carry, in which contestants pick up a stripped-down car from the ground and carry it across the finish line; and the Hercules Hold, where they stand between two soaring pillars, grip a handhold on each, and then hold the pillars upright, defying gravity for as long as possible, before their bodies surrender and the pillars tumble sideways on their hinges. We can all agree: These are some powerful dudes.

But they don't own the patent on strength.

❯❯ STRENGTH

Your capacity to exert and resist force; the force-producing quality of your muscle fibers; your ability to endure intense physical activity

Strength is a sport-specific concept, and successful athletes identify the metrics by which strength is defined in their own sport—and then train to get stronger.

Strength in weight lifting might mean a squat of 500 pounds (227 kg) and a power clean of 350 (159 kg). At the NFL combine, upper-body strength is tested by having players bench press 225 pounds (102 kg) as many times as possible, with a smattering of athletes able to better 40 reps. In baseball, strength might be determined by how far and fast you can throw a ball—or smack it with a bat. In soccer, a winger might be judged by top-end speed and stamina. In distance running, strength refers to an athlete's ability to maintain form and pace in the latter stages of a race. In basketball, it could mean endurance, vertical leap, or the ability to push your way through a defender. In volleyball, it can be the explosive lower-body force required to leap into the air and then the power to hold a block or spike the ball.

No matter the specific criteria for each sport, however, strength always arises from a singular attribute: an athlete's ability to exert force—or, if you're ever caught between two pillars in the Hercules Hold, to resist it.

WHAT'S STRENGTH?

Strength, for a speedster, is in many ways synonymous with speed itself. During acceleration, strength is a huge push during first-steps acceleration. During maximum velocity, it's the vertical force generated by hitting the ground hard and fast with each footstrike. But strength goes beyond generating speed. It also refers to the sturdiness and cohesion of the body (yours) producing the speed. Just as the X-1, the plane Chuck Yeager flew to first break the speed barrier on October 14, 1947, had been modeled after a .50-caliber machine-gun bullet and reinforced to absorb 18 times the force of gravity (18 Gs), you'll have to sculpt and reinforce your body for the following:

▸ **Stability:** Maintaining posture—or altering and then regaining it— during athletic movements that involve speed and agility

▸ **Injury prevention:** Strengthening muscles, both eccentrically and concentrically, to safely absorb, produce, and resist the forces encountered during practice and competition

▸ **Endurance:** Persevering until the play is finished or the sprint is won (more on speed endurance in Chapter 7)

Hammy Time

If your sport requires speed and agility—and almost all sports do—then your hamstrings are operating in the danger zone. If you've previously suffered a hamstring injury, then you've already got one foot in the infirmary. Hamstring injuries are the bane of sports.

  ▸ **NFL:** Hamstring strains account for 22 percent of all running back injuries, 14 percent of defensive back injuries, and 12 percent of wide receiver injuries (college football has similar rates).
  ▸ **Pro Soccer:** Hamstring injuries strike 12 percent of players and account for 17 percent of all injuries, as well as being the most common injury for soccer players at lower levels.
  ▸ **Professional Baseball:** Hamstring injuries account for 6 percent of all injuries and are the leading cause of time loss due to injury (approximately 25 days missed per injury).
  ▸ **Track & Field:** Hamstring strains account for 29 percent of sprinters' injuries.

The list goes on, with hamstring strains going viral in sports like tennis, rugby, skiing, judo, and bull riding—yes, bull riding! If you're running fast, changing direction, or otherwise putting torque to your thighs, you might as well paint a bull's-eye on your hammies.

With that in mind, here are some steps for safeguarding your hamstrings:

Step 1: Identify when hamstring strains are likely to occur

Late swing and early stance (i.e., braking) phases are the most dangerous parts of the gait cycle for hamstrings. In 1980, sprint research pioneer Dr. Ralph Mann branded early stance as the period when the magnitude of hip and knee activity placed the hamstrings most at risk. More recently, Chumanov, Heiderscheit, and Thelen, in a 2011 study, joined a chorus of opposing viewpoints, concluding that "the hamstrings are at greater risk for injury during the late swing phase of high-speed running." Chumanov et al. found that the hamstrings undergo eccentric contraction during—and only during—late swing and argued that hamstring injury is directly related to this type of contraction. A 2017 study staked out a middle ground, reporting that hamstrings encounter loads equal to 10 times body weight during late swing and eight times body weight during early stance. The study

>>

labeled the entire period the "swing-stance transition period" and concluded that risk factors for hamstring strain were high throughout the entire transition.

Step 2: Identify the risk factors that lead to hamstring strains

The swing-to-stance transition is when most hamstring strains occur, but there's disagreement over which risk factors precipitate the injuries. Here's what we know:

A 2008 study on elite male sprinters blamed weak same-side muscles for hamstring injuries. Another 2008 study following professional soccer players cited "strength imbalances between the hamstrings and quadriceps"—although 31 percent of athletes with recurrent injuries didn't have this imbalance.

Scar tissue from previous hamstring strains is often cited as a factor in reinjury. But a 2010 study—during which athletes ran at paces between 60 and 100 percent of maximum velocity—found no difference between scarred and unscarred hamstrings when it came to flexibility, strength, or muscle activation.

A 2017 study on amateur soccer players found the players' hamstring strains were correlated with weak glute and trunk muscle activation, joining numerous studies that have settled on "neuromuscular control" as the primary cause of injury.

The most-cited factor for hammy injuries is the high load incurred during the swing-stance transition, with the eccentric load of late swing seen as especially perilous.

All that said, a 2010 study on amateur soccer players that scrutinized player age, position, injury history, and performance level found only a single significant risk factor for hamstring injury: previous hamstring injury.

Therefore, the first rule of hamstring injury-prevention is: Don't injure your hamstrings.

Step 3: Identify the exercises that can prevent injury and reinjury

Two successful approaches to preventing and rehabilitating hamstring injuries are incorporated into the SpeedRunner system—because you can't be a speedster if you can't get off the couch.

Eccentric training. You place an enormous eccentric strain on your hamstrings during late swing. That makes it a no-brainer to strengthen your hamstrings eccentrically. A 2015 study on male soccer players found that performing Nordic Curls [page 202], an eccentric hamstring exercise, reduced hamstring injuries by two-thirds. A 2011 study on Danish pro soccer players again reported one-third the hamstring injury rate for

>>

athletes who performed Nordic curls. These results have been replicated in multiple studies. Some researchers, however, have objected to the Nordic curl routine on the basis that it only includes joint movement at the knee, while running causes hamstring strain at the knee and hip. These authors suggest adding exercises like the Single-Leg Deadlift (page 208) to eccentrically train the hamstring through hip movement, too.

Sprint and agility drills. A 2009 study assessed neuromuscular control in Australian Rules Football players. Believing poor neuromuscular communication to be a factor in hamstring injury, the authors put study participants through a HamSprint program—a mix of running drills, agility exercises, and explosive starts. The result was "significant improvement" in neuromuscular control and fewer hamstring injuries. Another 2009 study followed elite female soccer players for three years. These athletes also performed drills and exercises, and they reduced injuries by two-thirds, while missing only 10 percent as much playing time as their peers. Even more encouraging, a 2004 study compared a progressive agility and trunk stabilization (PATS) program—replete with multi-directional work, core strengthening, balance and proprioceptive training, and high-speed exercises—to a traditional stretching and strengthening hamstring rehabilitation routine. PATS athletes had a reinjury rate of 0 percent at one week and 7.7 percent at one year, while traditional rehab led to reinjury rates of 54.5 percent at two weeks and 70 percent at one year.

That makes for a pretty clear consensus. To combat hamstring injury, combine eccentric training with neuromuscular drills and exercises. Lucky for you, SpeedRunner does just that.

Step 4: Decide how long post-injury you should wait to begin rehab

Hamstring injuries lead to immediate pain, tenderness, swelling, and reduced range of motion. Before doing anything, you'll need to heal. That means 3 to 7 days for mild strain, and from two weeks to a month (or longer) for more severe injuries. Hamstring reinjury occurs at a rate of about 10 to 30 percent, and the long-term effects of the injury can last for up to two years. So be smart. And be patient. Of course, the best plan is to incorporate the SpeedRunner exercises that prevent hamstring injury before you get injured.

>> **SPECIAL STRENGTH**
Resistance work that incorporates similar joint movements as your sport but doesn't precisely replicate your sport's action (e.g., doing squats to improve first-steps acceleration); doing one type of training to improve strength in another type of training

Most athletes think better strength begins with building stronger muscles. It doesn't. It begins with your nervous system—with teaching your nervous system to better utilize the muscles you already have. During the early stages of training, nervous system adaptations are responsible for most strength gains. While your nervous system can stimulate strength gains in a single day, it will be 3 to 6 weeks before incremental gains in muscle-fiber size impact your bench press, squat, or 40-yard dash—and that much time again before those gains become substantial.

It shouldn't come as a surprise that your nervous system adapts so quickly. Think of how fast your nervous system adapts to various forms of stimuli. Jump into a cold lake or pool, and it takes only seconds for biting cold to transform into a manageable chill. Turn off the lights for bed, and within a couple minutes the pitch blackness softens. Put your hand on a table, and in no time its feel will begin to vanish from your conscious mind. While neuromuscular adaptation is different from involuntary sensory adaptation—neuromuscular strength adaptations result from self-motivated attempts to move your body more powerfully and efficiently—both types of nervous system adaptation begin within seconds, or less.

Muscle growth (called hypertrophy) also plays a role in strength gains. Obviously—just look at the biceps on those world's strongest men. But even in the beginning, when nervous system adaptations are king, microscopic muscle strengthening is crucial. When you train, muscle fibers break down and must be repaired. Damage untrained fibers too severely, and the result is DOMS (delayed onset muscle soreness), which causes debilitating pain and stiffness that can land you on the couch for a week.

In this chapter, we'll examine strength from several perspectives:

▸ **Muscles:** The components of muscles, different muscle fiber types, and the process of strengthening muscles
▸ **Nervous system:** The ways the nervous system adapts to create stronger muscle contractions and increased force
▸ **General, special, and specific strength:** Defining the objectives of each of these three approaches to strength training

► **Muscle by muscle:** A quick look at muscle groups that contribute to your performance, an explanation of their function, and exercises to strengthen each group

Strength development requires both nervous system and muscle group adaptation. Smart training pairs both to produce optimal strength gains.

LET'S TALK STRENGTH

WHILE STRENGTH, LIKE ROME, can't be built in a day, it can be improved overnight. And then improved more in a week. And even more in a month. "Strength" is an umbrella term that covers a multitude of sport-specific definitions. In the SpeedRunner system, we use "strength" to identify the muscular and nervous system adaptations you'll need to fortify speed, agility, and whole-body stability for athletic competition and improved fitness (i.e., there won't be any Olympic powerlifting). Let's start with a look at your muscles and nervous system.

Muscles

The human body has about 650 muscles. Your body contains three types of muscles: cardiac muscle, which is found in your heart; smooth muscle, which is involved with involuntary processes like digestion and blood pressure; and skeletal muscle, which is responsible for moving your body. SpeedRunner targets skeletal muscle, so let's break that down.

SKELETAL MUSCLE

Skeletal muscle accounts for one-third of your body mass, and it includes such Muscle Beach favorites as biceps, triceps, pectorals (chest), quadriceps, hamstrings, and calves. If a muscle helps move your body, it's a skeletal muscle. Skeletal muscle is composed of muscle fibers. Muscle fibers are clumped together in columns called fascicles. Fascicles are bound together to form muscles. And muscles can be organized into muscle groups—for example, your quadriceps muscle group consists of your rectus femoris, vastus lateralis, vastus medialis, and vastus intermedius. Don't worry about memorizing all those individual muscles. We'll discuss muscles by using their commonly recognized muscle group names (e.g., biceps and hamstrings).

SKELETAL MUSCLE FIBER TYPES

Muscle fibers can be further divided into three fiber types:

▸ **Slow-twitch (Type I):** These are your smallest fibers, and they contract the slowest and produce the least force. They also have amazing endurance—marathoners love them.
▸ **Intermediate fast-twitch (Type IIa):** These fibers are bigger and more powerful than slow-twitch fibers, but they possess less capacity for endurance.
▸ **Fast-twitch (Type IIx):** These are your biggest fibers, and they contract the fastest and produce the most force, even as they have almost no endurance—sprinters love them.

For maximum speed, agility, and strength, you'll need to recruit intermediate and fast-twitch fibers. These are the fibers responsible for the big push that begins acceleration, and they're the reason you can hit the ground hard and fast during top-end speed.

Each of your muscles contains all three fiber types. But all the fibers in each muscle don't have a single on-off switch. Instead, you recruit only as much muscle fiber as you need to exercise. When you exercise at low intensity, you recruit only slow-twitch fibers (and only as many as you need). As you exercise more intensely, you recruit intermediate fibers, too. At the greatest intensity—say, an overhead medball throw or an all-out sprint—you add fast-twitch fibers to the mix. You always recruit fibers from slow to fast, and any new fibers that you recruit are added to those already working—you don't replace working fibers, you reinforce them.

The SpeedRunner system manipulates the volume and intensity of your training to target specific muscle fibers in specific muscles. It's important that you follow the guidelines that accompany each exercise or drill. If you change volume and intensity, you change the workout.

STRENGTHENING MUSCLE

Let's turn up the magnification on our microscopes. Within each muscle fiber, there are smaller units called myofibrils. And within myofibrils are sarcomeres. And inside sarcomeres are protein myofilaments, including actin and myosin, which are 7 to 15 nanometers thick—a nanometer is one billionth of a meter. It's these tiny myofilaments that initiate muscle contraction. When myofilaments are weak, exercise damages them. Your body responds by rebuilding the myofilaments to be stronger than they were before and by adding new myofilaments. As your myofilaments get bigger and more numerous, your myofibrils split, forming more myofibrils, which makes your muscle fibers swell. When all the muscle fibers in a muscle get bigger (i.e., experience hypertrophy), people start complimenting you on your guns and six-pack. You find that you can run faster, jump higher, and lift heavy stuff. In short, you've gotten stronger.

67

STRETCHING YOUR MUSCLES

The SpeedRunner system doesn't include a stand-alone stretching routine, even though dynamic stretching (active movements that lengthen a muscle through its full range of motion) is built into many of the program's exercises and drills. Traditional static stretching—lengthening a muscle, then holding the position—leads to reductions in both strength (5 percent) and power (3 percent) in subsequent exercise. So Speed-Runner doesn't use it. "The way we work dynamically is completely different than how we might work statically," says Magness. "Carl Lewis [nine-time Olympic Gold Medalist in the sprints and jumps] couldn't touch his toes, yet watch him long jump and his dynamic range of motion is incredible."

Nervous System

Your nervous system comprises your brain, your spinal cord, and the nerves that stretch throughout your body. A nerve cell is called a neuron. You have approximately 85 billion of them in your brain and another billion of them in your spinal cord. Motor neurons send messages (called impulses) to your muscles, telling them to contract and relax. Sensory neurons receive stimuli detected by your senses. A single neuron can send up to a thousand messages per second, with each neuron directly connected to thousands of other neurons, passing signals via trillions of synaptic connections. Messages travel between 2 and 390 feet per second, depending on the type of nerve. All told, your entire nervous system can manage around 17 quadrillion connections per second. Yes, quadrillion. Your nervous system can crunch an enormous amount of data—as much as some of the largest supercomputers in the world. And it's ready, willing, and able to transform the training you perform into strength gains beginning on Day One.

MUSCLE FIBER RECRUITMENT

The intensity and volume of nervous system messaging determines which muscle fibers will be recruited and how long their contractions will last. Low-intensity messaging from your brain affects only smaller motor neurons in your spinal cord, the ones that control slow-twitch muscle fibers. Add intensity to the messaging, and you trigger larger motor neurons that control intermediate fibers. Send hair-on-fire messaging, and the largest motor neurons that control fast-twitch fibers are activated. What's more, if you keep sending messages to the same muscle fibers—like a burglar alarm that won't shut off—the fibers will contract more forcefully and for a longer period of time. "Intense" messaging doesn't mean furrowing your brow and squeezing shut your eyes. It means practicing that messaging through training until your nervous system learns how to recruit faster fibers at a sustained rate.

RECRUITMENT PATHWAYS AND MOTOR MODULES

As you practice for speed, strength, and agility (and for movements specific to your sport), your nervous system becomes quicker and more efficient at messaging for those tasks. In Chapter 1, we talked about motor modules—groups of muscles that are recruited in a sequence when performing athletic movements. We noted that fast learning occurred within seconds of initiating a new activity, even as slow learning required weeks. But your nervous system isn't limited to learning new motor module sequences. It also develops recruitment pathways at the micro level for muscle fibers themselves. How does that work? Consider the analogy of a postal carrier. On the first day of a new route, the carrier isn't sure which houses match which addresses, doesn't realize there are three houses down one driveway, and hasn't learned that the mailbox for one house is hidden behind a wall of shrubbery. As a result, delivery is slow. But a few days later, the carrier has the route down pat. Delivery is quicker, and all mail ends up at the right addresses. That's neuromuscular adaptation in a nutshell. Your nervous system learns the best pathways for recruiting the most effective muscle fibers within each muscle for an activity—then sequences the contraction of all muscles within a motor module for your strongest, most explosive performance.

IMMEDIATE STRENGTH GAINS

During the first weeks of training, almost all strength gains are achieved through adaptations in the nervous system. If you find that hard to believe, consider a 2004 meta-analysis on cross education. Cross education refers to training a muscle on one side of your body (e.g., your right biceps) and seeing strength gains appear in the opposite-side, untrained muscle (e.g., your left biceps). An average 7.8 percent strength gain in the untrained limb was reported—more than a third of the total gain recorded in the trained limb. The study concluded that "strength gains [in the untrained limb] do not result from changes in muscle." Can you guess where the strength gains came from? If you said, "the nervous system," you get a gold star. Nervous system adaptations are so effective that they carry over to untrained muscles.

REDUCED INHIBITION

One of the ways your nervous system increases contraction effectiveness is by relaxing muscles that oppose the contraction. Try flexing your biceps while simultaneously flexing your triceps. You can't do it. In a 2015 blog, physical therapist Robert Panariello, drawing on the work of Charlie Francis and Tudor Bompa, both coaches of Olympic gold medalists, wrote that "the highest skilled athletes are those with the ability to completely relax their antagonist muscle groups during high velocity movement." The effectiveness of a muscle's contraction depends on your nervous system's ability to turn off antagonist (opposing) muscles—or at least tone them down so that more powerful and efficient joint movements can occur.

LONG-TERM STRENGTH GAINS

Eventually, your muscles get bigger and stronger. You'll get "cut," maybe even "ripped." And as your muscle fibers get stronger, your nervous system has the option of recruiting fewer of them than previously required to do the same work—or all of them to perform more work. Let's say you own a business with 10 employees. You pay each employee $10 an hour. After a month, your employees' productivity increases by 100 percent. Five employees can do the work of 10. Now, you can either spend half as much money for the same work (by firing five employees) or get twice the work for the same payroll. It's win-win! It's the same with your nervous system. The same nervous system messaging now produces the same muscular power with fewer muscle fibers, or greater muscular power from the same number of fibers.

MAXIMUM MUSCLE ACTIVATION

Researchers use an instrument called an electromyogram to measure electrical activity in a muscle, then use that measurement to determine how strongly a muscle is contracting. During sprinting, contractions often exceed 100 percent of the predicted maximum voluntary contraction (MVC). It's tempting to explain away these super-contractions as the result of stretch-shortening cycles and stretch reflexes—both

>> **SPECIFIC STRENGTH**

Resistance work done while directly incorporating the joint movements and neuromuscular activation sequence of your sport—e.g., sled running to train for acceleration

of which are nervous system-driven and enhance contractions—but scientists Wiemann and Tidow found that sprinters generate muscle contractions greater than 100 percent MVC even when not influenced by these passive mechanisms. They concluded that your nervous system uses "higher discharge rates" and recruits muscle fibers that only "activate when running fast." In other words, you'll use some muscle fibers for sprinting that you won't use for other forms of exercise, at messaging rates that exceed normal nervous system behavior. That's an important point to remember as we head into strength training.

LET'S TALK STRENGTH TRAINING

THE SPEEDRUNNER PROGRAM focuses on strength training that is transferable to speed production, agility, and full-body stability. You will develop the kind of strength required for participation in most team sports while simultaneously targeting the injury-prevention exercises that will keep you healthy and ready to compete. Athletes who require increased bulk strength, such as American football players, might need to schedule extracurricular weight lifting sessions.

General, Special, and Specific Strength

You will perform three types of strength training while following the SpeedRunner system: general, special, and specific.

GENERAL STRENGTH

General strength exercises create overall body stability and fitness. The Plank (page 204), a basic core exercise, falls into this category. You've heard the proverb, "A chain is only as strong as its weakest link." Well, an athlete's body is only as strong as his or her weakest muscle, tendon, ligament, bone, or neural pathway.

SPECIAL STRENGTH

Special strength includes joint movements that you'll use in your sport—just not in the exact same way you'll use them in your sport. Weight Sled Marching (page 136) is an example of a special strength exercise for speed—you don't sprint, but you move your joints in a similar way while working a lot of weight. Coach, writer, and former NCAA All-American hammer thrower Martin Bingisser simplifies the concept to "strength you can apply to your sport." In other words, you engage in training that isn't exactly what you do in your sport, but which nevertheless improves your strength for what you do in your sport. Depth Jump (page 173), Hip Thrust (page 214), and Single-Leg Deadlift (page 208) are all exercises that lead to big gains in speed, even though none involves running.

SPECIFIC STRENGTH

Specific strength exercises follow the specificity of training principle: Athletes must train specific muscle fibers, muscles, and motor modules in the exact way that they'll be used during competition. Boyle defines specific strength as "movements with resistance that are imitative of the joint action." Weight Sled Run (page 138) is a good example of this because, even though you've increased resistance, you maintain at least 90 percent of your sprint speed, which preserves recruitment on the fiber, muscle, and motor module levels.

Muscle by Muscle

SpeedRunner strength training targets the main muscle groups responsible for speed and agility, as well as all-around core and upper-body strength. Eccentric strength exercises are specifically noted in entries for which they're available and appropriate, as eccentric training provides your best line of defense against injury, as well as preparing you for passive mechanisms like the stretch-shortening cycle.

ARMS AND UPPER BODY

While aggressive arm action plays a role in acceleration, that role is not well understood. During maximum velocity sprinting, your arms counterbalance the movements of your legs. That's basically it. A 2010 study found that arms contribute less than 1 percent of horizontal or vertical action. "Working" your arms creates tension in your muscles, and flexed muscles are harder (and take longer) to move than loose muscles. Instead, let your arms swing backward through their full range of motion. This triggers stretch reflexes in your chest and back muscles, which then propel your arms forward. On the other hand, during team-sports contests, you're rarely just sprinting. You'll need a combination of general and explosive strength in your chest, arms, shoulders, and back—the better to fend off opposing players, hang on to the ball, swing a bat, or perform any other action required in your sport.

72

Eccentric strength training: Push-Ups (page 222) are good for initial strengthening, then move up to Plyo Push-Ups (page 224) to target your chest's stretch-shortening cycle.

Strength training: To develop explosive, concentric upper-body strength, focus on exercises like Battle Ropes (page 218), Medball Push from Knees (page 221), and Plyo Push-Ups. For general upper-body and arm strength, perform Tug Rope with Weight Sled or Free Weight (page 217), Bear Crawl (page 196), and Crab Walk (page 197).

CALVES [includes gastrocnemius, soleus, and plantaris]

Your calves fire into action before initial contact, tensing in preparation for landing. They contract eccentrically during the braking phase as they undergo a powerful stretch-shortening cycle, then combine a strong concentric contraction with elastic recoil to propel you back into the air. How active are your calves? A 2005 study recorded their contraction strength at 174 percent MVC pre-footstrike, 189 percent MVC during braking, and 128 percent MVC during propulsion. Recall that 100 percent MVC is the maximum amount you can voluntarily contract your muscles (i.e., through isometric contraction). Additional research reported that across all running speeds, your calves contribute between 50 and 75 percent of the vertical force needed to accelerate your body upward, though at higher speeds the limited ground contact time negatively affects their ability to provide increased force. Important to any discussion of the calves is the role of the Achilles tendon, which is the greatest contributor to elastic recoil—not to mention a source of frequent injury (i.e., Achilles tendinitis and tendinosis).

Eccentric strength training: Heel Dips (page 230) develop stiffness in your Achilles tendon and help protect it from injury.

Strength training: We covered exercises for your calves (e.g., skipping drills, plyometrics, and ankle poppers) in previous chapters. No further training for stability and injury-prevention, beyond exercises in which the calves play a secondary role, is required.

CORE [includes pelvic floor muscles, rectus abdominis, obliques, and erector spinae, among others]

Your core is comprised of at least 29 muscles that stabilize your torso, spine, pelvis, and kinetic chain. They include abdominal muscles, paraspinal muscles, pelvic floor muscles, lower back muscles, hip girdle muscles, your diaphragm, and your glutes (tackled in the next entry). A 2012 article on running biomechanics, published in *Clinics in Sports Medicine*, stated that core muscles "help absorb and distribute impact forces and allow body movements in a controlled and efficient manner… They work in unison to allow breathing during running and the twisting motion required during the running cycle." That makes them pretty darn important.

Strength training: Athletes fall into two camps when it comes to core training: those who believe it's the holy grail of performance success and those who ignore it completely. SpeedRunner advises a Goldilocks approach: not too much, not too little, just the right amount. For core training, start with easier versions of exercises, then graduate to more challenging ones. Planks (page 204) become Plank Rotations (page 205), Bird Dogs (page 198) become Superman or Superwoman Planks (page 210), and Leg Lifts (page 200) prepare you for V-Ups (page 211). Exercises like Marching Bridge (page 201) and Windshield Wipers (page 212) help develop lower back and rotational stability.

GLUTES [includes gluteus maximus, gluteus medius, gluteus minimus, and tensor fasciae latae]

"The glutes can't get too strong in sports," says Bret Contreras, author of The Glute Guy website. "The stronger they get, the more powerfully they contract in sprinting and the better they protect against low back, knee, hamstring, and groin injuries." In previous chapters, we've talked a lot about the role of the glutes in hip extension, but they're also a powerful hip abductor—they prevent your torso from rotating forward with each stride as if you're a bow-legged cowboy pushing through a saloon's swinging doors. We'll address each glute function separately.

Glutes–hip extension

Beginning at knee lift position, your glutes contract concentrically to pull your thigh toward the ground. Once on the ground, the glutes provide powerful hip extension through midstance. Contreras notes that sprinting "activates 234 percent more mean gluteus maximus muscle than a vertical jump." In other words, your backside is working.

Eccentric strength training: Single-Leg Squat (page 207) and Single-Leg Deadlift (page 208) both include a controlled eccentric phase. Plus, Hip Thrust (page 214) can be transformed into a terrific eccentric exercise if you slow down (i.e., control) the lowering of your hips back to their start position.

Strength training: Concentric work began with weight sled exercises, plyometrics, and technique drills. For maximum glute activation, try the hip thrust exercise. It not only activates your glutes to 119 percent MVC, it also includes hip hyperextension, the key to speed.

Glutes–hip abduction

As hip abductors, your glutes contract to stabilize your pelvis during running, to move your leg sideways, and to rotate your thigh outward. Let's look at pelvis stability first. When you land on one leg, gravity tries to tug your opposite-side hip toward the ground. By contracting your glutes on the landing-leg side, you keep a level plane across your hips. Strong glutes also offset forward pelvic tilt, which is a speed-killer. And they prevent your hips from twisting and turning with each rotation of your arms and shoulders—good for Elvis, not so good for you. When you need to make a quick cut on the field or court, abductors move your leg sideways, and when you need to hurdle a defender who just fell down in your path, they rotate your thigh outward. Finally, your abductors are handy for keeping your knees from knocking into one another during forward sprinting.

Eccentric strength training: Your best bet is Side Steps with Resistance Band (page 227). Focus on controlling the movement of your trailing leg as you recreate your original stance from step to step. A good exercise to pre-train your abductors is Side Leg Lifts (page 206)—again, focus on controlling your working leg while you lower it.

Strength training: For general strength, Fire Hydrant (page 199) and Monster Walk (page 226) are great. For special strength, you can't beat Weight Sled Crossover (page 160). And for specific strength, Side Steps (Quick) (page 149) prepares you for competition-style, lateral agility.

HAMSTRINGS [includes semimembranosus, semitendinosus, and biceps femoris]

Your hamstrings just might be your most important sprinting muscle. According to Wiemann and Tidow, "hamstrings are singled out as the most important contributors to produce the highest speed levels." And Morin et al., in their 2015 study, write that "horizontal force production is predominantly determined by hamstring strength and end-of-swing level of activity [for hamstrings]." Your hamstrings help extend your hip after knee lift position, endure a load of up to 10 times your body weight while eccentrically controlling your lower leg before initial contact, endure up to eight times your body weight co-extending your hips during braking, and then hyperextend your hip during propulsion. As your speed increases, EMG results show that hamstring activity also increases—while glute and quadriceps activity remains constant or even declines.

Eccentric strength training: Eccentric contraction is so important to maximum velocity (to the stretch-shortening cycle that proceeds hammering the ground at initial contact) that you'll want to devote extra time to eccentric hamstring training for that reason alone. Also, this is the muscle group that speedsters injure the most, so you'll want to immunize it against injury. (See "Hammy Time," page 61, for a rundown on eccentric hamstring training.)

Strength training: As with glutes, your hamstring strength training was already in overdrive in the acceleration and maximum velocity chapters. Also as with glutes, the Hip Thrust (page 214), with its emphasis on hip hyperextension, is a great concentric exercise for your hammies.

HIP ADDUCTORS [includes adductor brevis, adductor longus, adductor magnus, pectineus, and gracilis]

Hip adductors, the muscles that bring your thighs together and rotate them inward, are active constantly during the gait cycle. During normal running, your adductors work with your abductors to keep your legs oriented forward. On the field or court, your adductors power the crossovers that allow you to change direction. When sprinting, your adductors fill another role. Wiemann and Tidow were among the first to argue that, during late swing, the adductor magnus helps your glutes and hamstrings with hip extension. As the adductor magnus's leverage changes near toe-off, it becomes a hip flexor, a role that continues until your swing knee passes under your hips, at which point it becomes a hip extensor again. It's believed that other adductors perform similarly.

Eccentric strength training: Adductor training is generally wrapped into exercises that target other muscles. That said, the lateral lunges you perform as part of the Lunge Clock (page 216) offer a good eccentric stimulus.

Strength training: Your adductors are activated during numerous exercises, without serving as a focal point (e.g., Squats, Lunges, Bear Crawls, and Windshield Wipers). For special strength, Weight Sled Crossover (page 160) can't be beat. For specific strength, Side Steps (Quick) (page 149) and Standing Starts (page 133) will prepare you for practice and competition.

HIP FLEXORS (includes iliopsoas, rectus, sartorius, tensor fasciae latae, pectineus, adductor longus, adductor brevis, and gracilis)

Your hip flexors lift your thigh—and hence, your knee. That's key for sprinting, but it's also important for agility. Quick footwork requires fast-acting flexion at your ankles, knees, and hips. While elastic recoil will keep your feet popping off the ground, your hip flexors will give you the knee lift required to make every move count.

Eccentric strength training: Two great exercises are already part of your core and quadriceps training: Leg Lifts (page 200) and Walking Lunges (page 176). For the former, control your legs as you lower them toward the ground. For the latter, "control" remains the operative word—maintain muscle tension as you both raise and lower your center of gravity.

Strength training: Mountain Climbers (page 203) specifically target your hip flexors. But you'll give this muscle group a good workout with agility ladder drills, cone drills, and technique drills, especially Bounding (page 127).

QUADRICEPS (includes rectus femoris, vastus lateralis, vastus medialis, and vastus intermedius)

Like your calves, your quadriceps spring into action during late swing in preparation for landing. They continue to fire through braking, when they absorb vertical force eccentrically, and then become less active during propulsion—they contribute to toe-off to end stance period, but most of propulsion is driven by elastic recoil. Illustrating just how little quadriceps contribute to propulsion, one key study recorded quadriceps activity of 159 percent MVC prior to initial contact, 130 percent MVC during braking, and only 33 percent MVC during propulsion. Of course, during acceleration, things are a little different. A big part of that huge push that launches you into acceleration comes from knee extension, and knee extension is driven by your quadriceps. As acceleration continues, the contribution from your quadriceps decreases, but that big push comes in handy any time you're cutting on a dime, or leaping into the air, or facing a competitor nose-to-nose, about to square off in the trenches.

> **Eccentric strength training:** Step-Downs (page 229) is a special strength exercise that helps prepare your quadriceps for the eccentric landing of each stride.

> **Strength training:** Air Squats (page 194) are a good primer for initial strengthening, and general strength work includes Walking Lunges, Lunge Clock, and Single-Leg Squats. Special strength is worked with Weight Sled Push, plyometrics, countermovement jumps, and hopping; and specific strength with Weight Sled Run, Hill Sprints, Push-Up & Sprint, and others.

TIBIALIS ANTERIOR

You probably haven't given much thought to your tibialis anterior; you may not even know which muscle it is. But it works so hard and so consistently during both speed and agility that it seems wrong to ignore it. Your tibialis anterior is located on the outside of your shin, and it's responsible for dorsiflexion, which means that it lifts your foot toward your shin. Research found that the tibialis anterior muscle has the highest sustained muscle activity in the ankle during the running cycle—more than your calves. You dorsiflex before landing, and then you dorsiflex again immediately upon toe-off (your body's way of making sure you don't scrape your toes on the ground during swing phase). Only at top-end speed, when knee flexion during swing guarantees good ground clearance, does your tibialis anterior ease up on its swing-phase dorsiflexion.

Strength training: You won't directly target your tibialis anterior. And you don't have to, as it plays a role in every exercise or drill in which your feet leave or land on the ground.

Whole-Body Strength

One shortcoming of training muscles in isolation is that you rarely use them that way in competition. Instead, you integrate contraction and relaxation of many muscles across multiple joints to create movement. That's the reason we run a stride after every technique drill—to integrate the isolated target of the drill (e.g., knee lift) into the full-body movement (e.g., sprinting) that represents our true training goal. For this reason, SpeedRunner includes exercises that recruit big contributions from both upper- and lower-body muscles, and which require your nervous system to control those muscles in a manner that produces the greatest force.

Strength training: Overhead Medball Throw (page 220) and Tug Rope with Weight Sled or Free Weight (page 217) both involve whole-body integration of muscles to create force. The Overhead Medball Throw teaches team-sports athletes the art of transferring power from the lower body to the torso and arms to augment upper-body force. Medball Push and Sprint takes this activity a step further, requiring a short sprint after launching the medball.

CHAPTER 5 FINAL WORD

Strength is a general term that athletes define according to the specific force requirements of their sport. For a speedster, strength includes lower-body explosive power to generate both a huge push during acceleration and a ground-shaking footstrike during maximum velocity. For a team-sports athlete, strength also implies the power to start, stop, and move laterally. Beyond basic speed and agility strength, the SpeedRunner system targets neuromuscular adaptations that create movement stability (i.e., posture and form) and structural stability (i.e. resistance to fatigue and injury). After completing your SpeedRunner strength training, your body—like Yeager's X-1 on that fateful October morning—will be ready for launch.

6

AGILITY, BALANCE, AND PROPRIOCEPTION

'll never forget the first time I saw Pelé perform a bicycle kick. It was August 1976, long before the United States soccer boom, and I was watching the New York Cosmos play the Miami Toros on TV. I knew nothing about professional soccer, but I knew this guy Pelé had been paid a then-astronomical sum of $2.8 million for three years to unretire and sell soccer to America. I was slumped on the couch, enjoying but not sold, when a lobbed cross pass triggered one of the most amazing athletic moves I've ever seen. As the pass angled down, Pelé turned his back to the goal, sprang into the air off his right foot, threw his head and shoulders backward as if launching into a back flip, drove his left knee skyward, then snapped his right leg up from where it hovered above the turf, smacking the soccer ball with his right foot and driving it over his body—and straight into the net for a score. It was the ultimate combination of agility, balance, and proprioception, all rolled into one, and goes a

>> **AGILITY**
Your ability to rapidly change direction; your ability to execute a quick change of velocity (i.e., speed & direction) in response to a stimulus

long way to explaining why Pelé is considered one of the greatest soccer players of all time—if not *the* greatest.

Agility, balance, and proprioception. In sports, you need the first, and you can't have the first without the other two. Every change in direction requires an ability to reassert postural control and stability (i.e., balance). Every turn of the gait cycle, swing of the bat, or kick of the ball demands an awareness of exactly where your limbs, extremities, and other body parts are positioned—in relation to one another and the ground—in a given moment (i.e., proprioception).

"We're all too slow," writes Tim Keown in a 2012 ESPN piece on the reaction times and quickness of superstar pro athletes, "but the best of the best have figured out how to compensate for nature's deficiencies. They've learned how to cheat science."

SpeedRunner doesn't require you to cheat science, but it does help you compensate for nature's deficiencies—the sluggishness of your side steps, the instability of your backpedal, and the slow reaction time of your brain to a stimulus.

Simply put, if you want to succeed in sports, you must improve your agility—and the balance and proprioception that make it possible.

WHAT ARE AGILITY, BALANCE, AND PROPRIOCEPTION?

AGILITY IS THE ABILITY TO CHANGE DIRECTION RAPIDLY—laterally, horizontally, vertically, or spinning 360s if that's what's required. Balance and proprioception are two processes that allow you to do that. You can't have agility without balance and proprioception.

Agility

Let's say you're carrying the ball in football—or dribbling it in soccer—and a defender charges into your path. What do you do? Assuming you don't lateral or pass the ball, you probably cut right or left. That's agility. We know it when we see it. But how, exactly, did you do it? After all, you don't have an automatic cut-left-or-right reflex. Instead, you saw the defender, processed that your route was blocked, and then (as you know from the last chapter on strength) initiated a nervous-system-controlled sequence of muscle fiber, muscle, and motor module activation to execute the cut. So yes, agility is your "ability to rapidly change direction." But it's much more than that. It's the ability

Agility by the Numbers

The following chart represents how a panel of experts from ESPN ranked various sports based on the level of agility (on a scale of 1 to 10) demanded by the sport. Also included (not in ranked order) are the ratings given based upon speed.

AGILITY RANKING BY SPORT

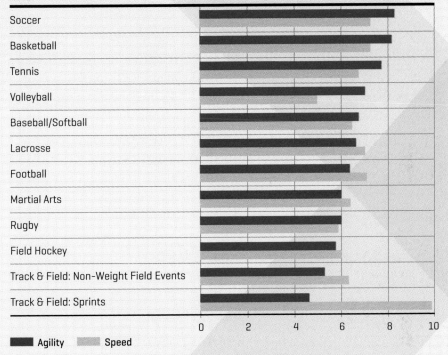

Of course, these rankings have limitations. For one thing, the panel ranked sports, not positions within sports. If the latter, there's no doubt that football's cornerbacks would set the standard among team athletes for both agility and speed. Or that basketball's less agile seven-footers might rank a few rungs down the ladder. Still, it offers a glimpse of how important agility is to competition—not to mention how interconnected it is with speed.

Information to create this chart was provided courtesy of espn.com.

to mentally process what you're seeing, initiate a hardwired sequence of muscle activation in response to what you're seeing, and utilize your balance and proprioceptive abilities to stay on your feet while changing direction. One other thing about agility: At its most basic, it represents a change in velocity (i.e., a change in speed, direction, or both). What else represents a change in velocity? That's right: acceleration. Agility is a multi-directional version of acceleration.

Balance

Before we discuss balance, we need to talk about your senses. Specifically, the fact that you don't have just five of them. You have maybe nine. Or 21. Experts disagree. The myth of five senses can be traced to Aristotle, who devoted five chapters in his c. 350 B.C. treatise *De Anima* to vision, hearing, touch, smell, and taste. Unfortunately, Aristotle's counting came up short. For instance, your sense of balance is generally considered a non-Aristotelian addition. For a quick demonstration of balance, do this: Stand up, and then slowly tilt forward. You'll quickly become aware of a force that you can't see, hear, touch, smell, or taste. It's called gravity, and you apprehend it through your sense of balance. Balance mixes sensory input from several sources: your inner ear, your eyes, and, in a preview of our next entry, your sense of proprioception, with which you track your body's position in space. Using this information, balance keeps your body upright and steady. That's important. Balance isn't *just* sensing. It's also reacting. It controls postural stability. It allows you, as an athlete, to run, cut, side step, backpedal, and land a jump without toppling to the ground.

Proprioception

I'm currently using proprioception to write this chapter. That's because I'm using my fingers to type without looking at my keyboard. Proprioception is your awareness of where all the parts of your body are located relative to one another and to the outside world. It doesn't require seeing those parts, just sensing them. Pelé exercised extraordinary proprioception during his bicycle kicks. He'd launch himself into the air, eyes on the soccer ball, while remaining perfectly cognizant of where his legs were in relation to the ball, where his body was in relation to the ground, how to use that knowledge to smack the ball into the goal, then land safely on the turf. For your own quick experiment in proprioception, close your eyes, then touch your right forefinger to the tip of your nose. Did you do it? If so, that's proprioception.

CHAPTER PREVIEW

IN THIS CHAPTER, we'll discuss the contributions of agility, balance, and proprioception to your athletic performance and overall fitness, and we'll explore ways to improve those contributions:

- ▸ **Breakdown:** How each skill relates to performance
- ▸ **Trainability:** Some of the obstacles faced when training agility
- ▸ **Exercises and drills:** How SpeedRunner addresses agility, balance, and proprioception training

For team-sports participants, these skills are non-negotiable. But even sprinters need agility to get out of the blocks. Sprinters also need highly tuned balance and proprioception to maintain stability at high speeds and to stay in their lanes, especially when navigating curves.

⟩⟩ BALANCE

Your ability to maintain your center of mass over your base of support (i.e., the area between your feet when you're standing); in dynamic balance, you must maintain stability and control as your body moves through space; your sense of gravity

LET'S TALK AGILITY

IN THEIR 2006 REVIEW OF STUDIES ON "AGILITY," Sheppard and Young determined that "no agreement of a precise definition of agility within the sports science community exists." So Sheppard and Young decided to create one. They proposed that agility be viewed as "a rapid whole body movement with change of velocity or direction in response to a stimulus." That's a good working definition to keep in mind as we talk about agility in this chapter.

The next step in discussing agility is identifying the factors that affect its execution. A 2015 review of 42 studies on agility in team sports identified three main factors that influence agility:

▸ **Cognitive and perceptual factors:** These include mental aspects, such as your ability to perceive the need to act, the length of time you spend deciding whether to act, the delay before you're able to implement action, and the outcome of your chosen course of action.
▸ **Technique factors:** These refer to skills (e.g., side-stepping, backpedaling, juking, etc.) that can be improved through preplanned workouts including drills and exercises.
▸ **Physical factors:** These are your physical attributes, such as acceleration and strength, although some, like your percentage of each muscle fiber type, are mostly innate. Any agility you display on the field or court will draw upon multiple physical components (e.g., your nervous system, muscle groups, and elastic recoil).

When discussing agility as it relates to athletic performance, there are two things about the above list to keep in mind:

1/ Cognitive and perceptual factors, for all their value, require only a fraction of the execution time as your subsequent physical action. In other words, your overall quickness depends more on action and less on the thinking that precedes it. That said, the success of any action depends almost entirely on your decision-making. A juke on the field that sends you straight into a defender's arms counts as an undesirable use of agility, no matter how quickly you execute the move.
2/ While technique can be improved dramatically through training, real-life competition doesn't perfectly mimic preplanned exercises and drills. For example, you rarely run agility ladder drills while a defender attempts to knock you on your can.

The bottom line is that agility is an extraordinarily complex combination of mental and physical factors, some trainable, some innate—all of which work together to produce the kinds of split-second actions and reactions that define top athletes.

LET'S TALK BALANCE

IT'S ONE THING TO BALANCE ON TWO FEET while standing in line at a bookstore, waiting to purchase *SpeedRunner* at the next available cashier's station. It's another to be a player on the field, balancing as you decelerate from a 20-yard sprint, plant one foot, bend at the knee to lower your center of mass, twist at the waist to direct your cut, perform a quick crossover, and then explode laterally, sprinting in a new direction. Without balance, it'd be impossible to attempt such a move—one where your center of mass is like a rubber ball bounced furiously via elastic string during an intense game of paddleball. On the field or court, balance both keeps you on your feet and ensures stability as you accelerate your center of mass in a new direction. Not only is that a difficult assignment, it's one your nervous system simply can't handle without proper preparation. It doesn't even try.

One 2013 study had runners perform short strides before cutting 90° laterally on a moveable platform. After 10 repetitions, during which the platform remained stable, the researchers caused the platform to wobble on the 11th rep. The result was that the runners' key stabilization muscles (e.g., the hamstrings and glutes) showed reduced activation. That's right: Even though the need for stabilization increased, the runner's nervous system and muscles helped out less. What happened? With no prior training for this specific challenge, the runners' ability to balance short-circuited. It froze. The study's authors suggest that our human nervous systems "might not be able to counteract instantaneously to threats [like this disruption of balance] by means of muscular recruitment in non-trained subjects."

The message is clear: If you want to maintain good balance while competing in your sport, you'll need to train for any sport-specific moves that might involve balance. That will require practice for two types of balance:

▸ **Static balance:** Maintaining balance while standing still
▸ **Dynamic balance:** Maintaining stability and control as you move

As with agility, there is no uniformly recognized definition of "balance." But you'll know it when you sense it—or, perhaps, especially when you don't.

85

LET'S TALK PROPRIOCEPTION

BECAUSE PROPRIOCEPTION IS SO IMPORTANT, allowing you to instantaneously track your hands, feet, arms, legs, and other body parts, it's processed over the fastest nerves in your body, nerves that can relay messages at 390 feet per second. Proprioceptive nerves are located in your muscles, tendons, and ligaments. They sense changes in position and relay them back to your central nervous system. Your central nervous system responds by sending commands to your muscles, which trigger contractions to maintain or change those positions. Proprioception governs everything from hand movements to stride length, from your ability to put on a shirt to your skill at driving a car. It's what makes it possible for you to swing a tennis racket, throw a football, spike a volleyball, or sink a basketball without staring at your hands while you perform the task. How important is proprioception to success in sports? A 2013 study on 100 elite athletes in various sports found that "30 percent of the variance in the sport competition level an athlete achieved could be accounted for by ... proprioceptive sensitivity scores for the ankle, shoulder, and spine [combined with] the number of years of sport-specific training." The authors conclude that while physical and mental preparation for sports is crucial, "proprioceptive ability is also an important determining attribute."

≫ PROPRIOCEPTION

Your awareness of your body's position and movement in space; your ability to track and manipulate all parts of your body—limbs, torso, the whole kit and caboodle—relative to one another and your surroundings

LET'S TALK AGILITY, BALANCE, AND PROPRIOCEPTION TRAINING

NOW THAT WE'VE DISCUSSED agility, balance, and proprioception's contributions to athletic performance, it's time to talk training. You'll be happy to know that any time you're training agility, you're also training balance and proprioception. They're as inseparable as the Three Musketeers—"All for one and one for all!" You might be less happy to know that there are dozens of different training approaches for agility. How do you pick the right one for you? Let's narrow down the choices.

- **Perceptual training:** Athletes use video clips to improve perceptual and decision-making skills. While watching video clips of actors performing agility moves on the screen, athletes perform the same drills. A 2011 study on rugby players found that perceptually trained athletes "improved significantly" in perception, response, and total agility time.

- **Human training:** Athletes respond to human commands or to movements by coaches and other participants. Some of the movements are deceptive (i.e., feints). In theory, this type of training should transfer directly to competition, where unplanned movements dominate. As Sheppard et al. explain in their 2006 paper on agility testing, "Open skills [i.e., reaction to a stimulus] cannot be pre-planned, whereas closed skills, such as sprint running or pre-determined changes of direction, can be pre-planned."

- **Small-sided games:** Teams with 1 to 3 players per side square off in miniaturized versions of full-scale competition. Advocates for this type of training consider it "an effective method of simultaneously training the physical, technical, and tactical qualities of a player."

- **Change-of-direction training:** This is basic physical and technique training. Athletes perform pre-planned cone drills, agility ladder drills, footwork drills, and alternative gaits (e.g., side steps and backpedaling) that mimic expected game-time movements.

The SpeedRunner system doesn't include the first three types of training listed above. First, SpeedRunner is designed to work as a program for athletes without access to training partners—that doesn't mean you can't work out with a partner (in fact, SpeedRunner encourages you to do so, and includes some partner exercises toward that end)—just that you should be able to perform the workouts on your own. Second, most athletes don't haves the set-up or support team to create the video tools for perceptual training. Third, there's no guarantee these training methods translate to better performance on the field or court. The best way to prepare for exactly what you'll face in your sport is to practice and compete in your sport.

SpeedRunner provides you with the fundamental skills you'll need, when the time comes, to master your sport-specific training. For agility, that means change-of-direction training. A 2013 study on youth soccer players found that a speed and agility program was "an effective way of improving agility, with and without the ball, for young soccer players." And a 2014 study comparing the benefits of change-of-direction training to small-sided games and a control group concluded, "Improvements in sprint, agility with ball, COD [change of direction], and jumping performance were higher with CODG [change-of-direction-trained athletes]."

SpeedRunner change-of-direction training includes:

▸ Cone drills
▸ Agility ladder drills (and no-props alternatives)
▸ Alternative gait training

You'll develop the neuromuscular control required for change-of-direction movement laterally, horizontally, and vertically—and you'll learn to execute that movement using multiple gaits.

Cone Drills

Cone drills target multiple aspects of agility: acceleration, deceleration, lateral and horizontal force production, posture adjustment, body mechanics, and, naturally, balance and proprioception. You'll change direction on a dime, transition between different gaits, and utilize multiple techniques and postures to navigate the various courses. Cone drills aren't about top-end speed. They're about controlled acceleration and deceleration, coupled with changes in direction meant to mimic the movements you'll make during competition. For acceleration-deceleration in all gaits, try the 20-Yard Square and 40-Yard Square (page 154). For practicing your jukes, there's the Figure 8 Drill (page 156), W-Pattern Cone Drill (page 158), and one of your metrics tests, the 3-Cone Drill (page 190). For a more explosive challenge, try Mini-Suicides (page 151) or another of your metrics tests, the 20-Yard Shuttle (page 188).

Agility Ladder Drills and No-Props Alternatives

Agility ladder drills are for footwork. Footwork provides the dynamic foundation for jukes, lateral cuts, gait transitions, and other agility moves. It's a good idea to walk through each new drill before attempting it. Then try it at half-speed. Then gradually increase your speed—if you start missing ladder spaces, start over and slow down. For improving basic foot speed, use Agility Ladder 3 Quick Steps (page 144) or, if you don't have access to an agility ladder, 3-Step, 1-Step (page 148). For simple horizontal foot-work practice, use either Agility Ladder Step In 'n' Out (page 146) or its no-prop alter-native, the Step Back 'n' Forth Drill (page 147). For lateral development, perform the Agility Ladder Ickey Shuffle (page 145)—as a no-prop alternative, mimic the footwork using a centerline as your guide. Finally, for those with a ladder, Agility Ladder 1-Legged Hops (page 140) and Agility Ladder 2-Legged Hops (page 142) help develop the strength you'll need to power many of the quick moves required on the field or court.

Alternative Gait Exercises and Drills

If you haven't done a lot of side-stepping or backpedaling, you'll need to practice both. Practice will help you develop the stability required to stay on your feet (e.g., if some-one shoves you while you're side-stepping). Backward Running (page 150) will train you to move fast in reverse without resorting to an out-of-control bound. Side Steps (Quick) (page 149) will teach you to move sideways rapidly, minus the "hop" between steps that results in reduced stability. One other piece of advice on gait: During agility drills, experiment with your gait for *forward* running. Most athletes prefer to move with a lower center of mass, less knee flexion, and lower knee lift while showing off their moves on the field or court. Find what works best for you.

Balance-and-Proprioception-Specific Training

A 2011 review of studies on balance ability and athletic performance concluded that "gymnasts tended to have the best balance ability," followed by soccer players, swim-mers, and basketball players. Of course, it shouldn't come as a surprise that the sports in which balance plays the biggest role are also the sports in which participants can balance the best. If you want to get better at balance, practice it.

SpeedRunner offers a steady diet of training that includes elements of both balance and proprioception—exercises such as Side Steps, Ankle Poppers, Walking Lunges, Air Squats with the Medball, the Lunge Clock, the Single-Leg Squat, the Superman or Superwoman Plank, and more. As we discussed earlier, you can't train agility *without* training balance and proprioception, so you'll get a great workout for all three skills with cone and agility ladder drills.

You'll also want to include Balance on 1 Leg (page 152) in your program. It's a simple exercise that serves as a good defense against ankle sprains. Ankle sprains are the most common injury in high school sports, accounting for roughly one in six injuries. And they're epidemic across all age groups, with the American College of Sports Medicine (ACSM) reporting 25,000 ankle sprains per day for Americans. The ACSM also reported that one of the major risk factors for ankle sprains is "impaired balance/postural control." Luckily, that's an easy problem to fix. A 2006 study followed football players who balanced on each foot for five minutes, five days a week, for four weeks during preseason. During the season, they suffered 77 percent fewer sprains than players who didn't perform the routine. It's a simple exercise, but it's effective.

CHAPTER 6 FINAL WORD

When you improve your agility, balance, and proprioception—and when you then add those skills to your upgraded acceleration and maximum velocity—you become a better athlete. You're faster, stronger, and quicker. That may not translate to a Pelé-like bicycle kick. But at a minimum, you are a highly functioning athlete, a true Speed-Runner, on your way to becoming the competitor you're meant to be. And about that bicycle kick—never say never....

7

ENERGY SYSTEMS AND SPEED ENDURANCE TRAINING

Your car runs on gasoline. Your barbecue runs on propane. Your refrigerator runs on electricity. Pioneer wagon trains were fueled by horsepower. There was even a Formula 3 racecar in Coventry, England, that ran on 30 percent biodiesel derived from vats of Cadbury chocolate.

But what about you?

When you're sprinting and changing direction, what powers you?

If you answered "ATP," go to the head of the class.

There are a lot of misconceptions about how humans produce energy. Most of us know that the food we eat is related to the energy we produce. Fewer of us understand that carbohydrates, fats, and proteins are just raw materials from which we create our actual energy source, ATP. A good analogy is crude oil, a raw material that's processed at refineries to produce gasoline (and diesel, kerosene, jet fuel, motor oil, and grease,

---

》 ENERGY SYSTEMS

Three pathways used by your body to convert carbohydrate and fat (and sometimes protein) into ATP, the only energy your muscles can use

---

Sprint Fuel

When you initiate a sprint—or any other all-out lift, push, jump, juke, or athletic movement—your phosphagen system kicks into gear within thousandths of a second, responding twice as quickly as your other anaerobic system, the "fast glycolysis" pathway of the glycolytic system (what most athletes think of when they discuss anaerobic energy). Until your phosphagen system revs up, you use stored ATP as your fuel source. Aerobic energy lags behind, but will eventually produce massive amounts of energy—the delay in producing aerobic energy results from the 30 to 40 seconds it takes for your cardiovascular system to deliver an increased supply of oxygen to the affected muscle fibers.

ENERGY SYSTEM CONTRIBUTION TO SPRINTING

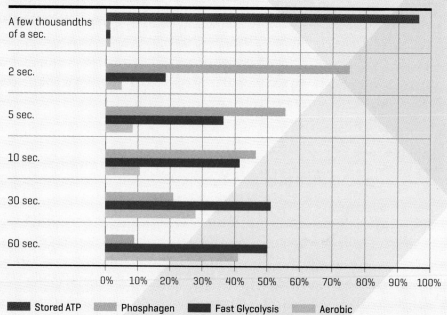

This chart represents average values recorded when athletes' energy systems fuel a sprint (or other all-out effort). There will be variance among athletes based on gender, percentage of muscle fiber types, fitness, etc. Also, the *total* amount of energy you produce at any moment will vary over the course of the sprint/activity—this chart represents the percentage of total energy at six intervals. Still, it gives you a good idea of how your energy systems combine to fuel maximum efforts.

not to mention floor wax, tires, shampoo, toilet seats, hand lotions, panty hose, lipstick, toothbrushes, and much more).

There are commercial products that promise "energy"—like 5-Hour Energy, Red Bull, and Monster Energy—when all they're really peddling are stimulants. Sure, they'll stop you from getting drowsy and delay fatigue, but they don't contribute much actual energy. For example, 5-Hour Energy has four calories, enough to power a 150-pound (68 kilogram) man or woman through a leisurely 80-yard walk or 60 yards of fast running. Eight ounces of Red Bull has 100 calories, the same as a small banana. And a 16-ounce Monster Energy drink has 210 calories, which will fuel our 150-pound person for nearly 2 miles of running—not bad until you consider that a good soccer player runs 5 to 6 miles in a single match.

As a speedster in team or individual sports, your ability to perform is directly related to your ability to produce energy quickly and efficiently. That's how you fuel a sprint, change of direction, push, pull, throw, hit, spike, block, lift, shot, or shove that knocks an opponent on his or her keister. You already know how to eat. Now, your body needs to learn the art of rapid fueling. In an arena where a tenth of a second can make the difference between success and failure, the ability to produce high-octane fuel in less than that tenth of a second is essential.

WHAT ARE ENERGY SYSTEMS?

YOUR MUSCLES GET THEIR ENERGY from one source: the molecule ATP. Your energy systems have one job: to produce ATP. You eat food because it contains energy—calories—in the form of carbohydrates, fats, and proteins. But you don't directly use the calories from food. Instead, you use your energy systems to convert those calories into a different form of energy—the energy found in the molecule adenosine triphosphate (ATP), which can then be used to power your muscles. Think of it as going to a casino in Las Vegas. You bring wads of cash, but you don't use it to bet double zero in roulette or to double down in blackjack. You use it to buy chips at the table or a cashier's cage. Then you use those chips to bet. When it comes to powering your muscles, ATP molecules are your chips.

You have three energy systems:

▸ **Phosphagen system:** An anaerobic system that uses creatine phosphate to create ATP

▸ **Fast glycolysis:** An anaerobic system that uses carbohydrates (in the form of glycogen and glucose) to create ATP

▸ **Aerobic system:** A system that uses carbohydrates, fats, and oxygen to create ATP

Your anaerobic and aerobic systems don't operate separately, with one turning on when another turns off. All three energy systems are *always* working. It's just that each system has unique characteristics that make it the primary contributor of ATP depending on the intensity and duration of the activity. We'll discuss this more shortly. For now, understand:

1/ All three energy systems are always "on."
2/ All three systems produce ATP.
3/ ATP is the only energy source your muscles use.

The difference between aerobic and anaerobic energy is simple. Aerobic energy production requires oxygen. Anaerobic energy production doesn't. That's it. Sure, that's a *big* difference, and it's not the only difference in the way each pathway produces energy. But as far as "aerobic" and "anaerobic" are concerned, it's all about the oxygen.

LET'S TALK ENERGY SYSTEMS

ATHLETES ARE SOMETIMES SURPRISED to hear that they use aerobic energy in sprints as short as 100 yards—up to 20 percent aerobic energy (with top speedsters closer to 10 percent). Likewise, endurance runners are often shocked to discover that the first 30 to 40 seconds of their runs and races are the most anaerobic. But until your lungs, heart, and blood can deliver more oxygen to your muscle fibers, a process that takes 30 to 40 seconds, increased aerobic energy production remains on hold. In the meantime, your anaerobic energy production fills the gap. Here's another misconception: Athletes tend to believe that sprinting 50 yards uses more calories than jogging the same distance. It doesn't. You burn the same number of calories. It's just that you use your energy systems differently to create that fuel.

As an athlete, you'll want to increase your energy systems' efficiency, output, and rate of output. You'll also want to focus on the energy systems you tap the most. An

NFL running back won't need to develop the aerobic system of a cross-country runner. But a soccer player must develop *all* of his or her energy systems, given that soccer mixes sprints with endurance.

ATP

ATP has been called the "common currency" of energy. No matter what you're doing—sprinting, shooting free throws, or sitting on the couch—you're using ATP to do it. At any given moment, you maintain a reserve of approximately 100 grams of ATP. That's enough to fuel a few minutes of watching TV or a few seconds of intense exercise. During a normal day, you'll recycle every molecule of ATP about 500 to 700 times. Train hard, and you might double that. In sports, your first step, jump, push, pull, or other athletic action depletes your ATP to a level that immediately triggers a five-alarm response. If this were Gotham City, Commissioner Gordon would shine the bat-signal into the sky. And while your body isn't Gotham City, your energy systems, and one in particular, make like Batman and come to the rescue.

Phosphagen System

A few thousandths of a second after you start exercising, your phosphagen system kicks into high gear. Using a small store of intra-muscle creatine phosphate (CP), this system cranks out energy twice as quickly as your next-fastest responder, fast glycolysis. Your phosphagen system arrests the decline of intra-muscle ATP, stabilizing levels at 80 percent of normal. The only problem? It's a short-lived system, with your muscles capable of banking only limited stores of CP. You'll get a great 10 seconds, but by 12 to 20 seconds into your effort, you'll be running on CP fumes. Afterward, it will take about three minutes to replenish your CP stockpile.

 ATP
A molecule that provides the energy for all muscle contractions; the end product of aerobic and anaerobic energy production

Fast Glycolysis

As the phosphagen system fades, fast glycolysis (part of your glycolytic system and an anaerobic process) takes over as your primary ATP supplier. The centerpiece of this system is a multi-step chemical reaction, called glycolysis, which takes place within your muscle fibers. Glycolysis breaks down carbohydrates (in the form of glucose or glycogen) to quickly produce 2 to 3 ATP molecules plus two pyruvate molecules. These molecules can either jump-start a fresh round of glycolysis or find a nearby mitochondrion (an aerobic energy-producing factory within your muscle fibers) to initiate aerobic energy production. If there's limited oxygen in your muscle fibers (because your blood has yet to deliver an increased supply), then back to glycolysis it is. This fast glycolysis cycle will spin round and round, churning out a huge supply of ATP while it lasts, which it does for approximately 1 to 2 minutes at maximum capacity—or indefinitely during less intense exercise. Here's what you should know about fast glycolysis: First, it's your primary ATP-producing system between 10 seconds and a minute of all-out effort; second, any time you run faster than 3K-race pace, you *must* supplement your aerobic energy production with ATP supplied by this system (your aerobic system can't produce enough energy on its own to fully fuel intense efforts).

Aerobic System

Aerobic energy is produced within each muscle fiber's mitochondria. You have between hundreds and thousands of mitochondria (microscopic structures, each a few micrometers long) floating inside the gel-like universe of each muscle fiber, and they produce *all* your aerobic energy. To do so, they break down carbohydrates and fats to create ATP. If you're walking or running, your pace determines the percentage of ATP produced from each raw energy source:

- **Walking:** 15–20% carbohydrate, 80–85% fat
- **Distance run:** 40–55% carbohydrate, 45–60% fat
- **Tempo pace:** 60–70% carbohydrate, 30–40% fat
- **5K/10K race:** 80–90% carbohydrate, 10–20% fat
- **Sprint:** 100% carbohydrate

Tempo pace is defined as "comfortably hard"; it's faster than a distance run but slower than a 10K. Some team-sports athletes (e.g., soccer) might use this effort to transition from offense to defense or for other sub-maximal running during practice and competition.

While glucose or glycogen (carbohydrates) net you only 2 to 3 ATP during fast glycolysis, those same molecules will net you 32 to 33 ATP during aerobic energy production. And a single fatty acid processed aerobically can net up to 129 ATP—unfortunately, processing fat requires so many steps (and so much time to perform those steps) that it's not useful for fueling intense efforts. All athletes benefit from some aerobic training. Sprinters prize aerobic adaptations for recovery and long sprints. Athletes in sports like soccer and basketball—sports with an endurance component—generate most of their ATP aerobically during practice and competition.

Elastic Recoil

No, this isn't an energy system. It's just a reminder that about half the energy you use during each running stride is provided by elastic energy. If you want to improve your energy systems, start by improving elastic recoil, which decreases your energy systems' required contributions.

Speed Endurance

You're only as fast as the amount of energy you can produce. And you can only sustain "speed" while you continue producing enough energy. In the sidebar "Sprint Fuel" (page 92), you'll notice that, within seconds, all three energy systems increase ATP production, working together to provide the surge in energy you need to sprint (or to perform other high-intensity activities). "Speed endurance" is your ability to keep all three energy systems cranking out ATP for as long as possible. Again, more energy equals more speed. To improve speed endurance, you'll need to identify the trainable aspects of each system.

> **Phosphagen system:** By itself, this system can't generate enough ATP to fuel even 10 seconds of sprinting. But by increasing creatine phosphate stores, you can extend this system's contribution. And boosting the volume of enzymes available to break down CP speeds up energy production. Creatine supplements are an easy way to increase CP by up to 20 percent.

> **Fast glycolysis:** Increasing the rate at which this system produces ATP makes it more valuable during acceleration, when the phosphagen system does most of the heavy lifting, and later will extend the time you can remain

Speed for Distance Runners

In my decades of coaching, writing about running, and competing in races from 400 meters to the half-marathon, I've noticed one universal characteristic of distance runners: We can turn any workout—I mean *any workout*—into a distance run. Tell distance runners to do hill sprints, and we'll jog 400 yards between reps. Ask us to train in the weight room, and we'll tag 5 miles on afterward. And that's a problem. Because turning those workouts into distance runs negates most of their value, and because speedwork and resistance training are essential for running your best.

Exercise scientist Tim Noakes, MD, in his *Lore of Running* (considered the bible of distance running research), notes that "the ability to produce force rapidly when the foot is on the ground, thereby maintaining a short ground contact time, is a factor predicting 5-km running time," and that "explosive-type strength training may improve running performance as a result of neuromuscular adaptations." He later concludes that "the fastest athletes in endurance events of 5 km or longer tend also to be faster over the short distances from 100 m to 1500 m." A 2016 meta-analysis looked at studies involving high-level middle- and long-distance runners whose training included lower-body resistance exercises, plyometrics, and short sprints. The study's authors concluded that this high-intensity training "showed a large, beneficial effect." They recommended a "strength training program including low to high intensity resistance exercises and plyometric exercises performed 2 to 3 times per week." Sound familiar? If not, go back and read Chapters 2 through 6 of this book.

I've personally used resistance training, plyometrics, hills, drills, and sprints since I began competing as a masters distance runner in 2002. In the interim, I've set American 5K age group records for men's 45–49 (14:34), 50–54 (15:02), plus 55–59 (15:42), as well as accumulating age-group records at other distances and six USA masters XC overall individual titles.

Bottom line: If you're a distance runner who isn't training strength and speed, you're getting beaten by a distance runner who is.

›› SPEED ENDURANCE

The ability to accelerate or perform at maximum velocity repeatedly during competition; the ability to prolong the time spent at near-maximal speed at near-maximal speed. For team-sports athletes, this is the system that you'll tap most for repeated sprints and high-intensity movements. Increasing anaerobic enzymes and developing "buffering" systems against the fatigue-inducing byproducts of fast glycolysis are both legitimate targets for training.

Aerobic system: Although this system contributes less energy to sprints and high-intensity activities, it remains an essential energy contributor to both. It accounts for 3 to 10 percent of the energy required for acceleration, and it's the primary system used during sub-maximal running and recovery. It's also the system with the most potential for improvement—you can literally double its energy output with smart training.

Whether your goal is an extended sprint or the ability to maintain speed and power during repeated sprints, speed endurance is essential to your performance. Gassers 30/30 (page 183) is the only speed endurance training included in the SpeedRunner schedules. But don't panic. There's a supplemental workout plan provided at the end of this chapter.

LET'S TALK ENERGY SYSTEMS TRAINING

THE SPEEDRUNNER SYSTEM doesn't make energy system training a focal point, but that doesn't mean your energy systems aren't being trained. With every exercise, drill, repetition, and manipulated recovery interval, you're training your phosphagen and fast glycolysis systems. Just as football players might need extra time in the weight room, however, most team-sports athletes will need some speed endurance training to ensure their best performance.

Enzymes and Efficiency

Your ability to maximize your energy systems rapidly and efficiently depends largely on each system's enzymes. Enzymes are molecules that accelerate chemical reactions, such as those involved in energy production. One 2001 study concluded, "Enzyme adaptations represent a major metabolic adaptation to sprint training, with enzymes of all three energy systems showing signs of adaptation to training." For your phosphagen system, enzyme training requires short, fast sprints or other high-intensity efforts (e.g., Jump Squats, Plyo Push-Ups, and Mini-Suicides), with 2 to 3 minutes recovery time. For fast glycolysis, the duration of your repetitions will have to be longer—about 20 to 40 seconds (like the repetitions featured in this chapter's "Speed Endurance Training" table, page 102). The 2001 study reported that enzyme levels for both your phosphagen and fast glycolysis systems will remain stable for 2 to 6 months post-training (assuming some continued sports-related activity), meaning that the endurance you develop during your SpeedRunner training will last through your competitive season. For aerobic enzymes, aerobic system-based workouts, represented by the 30-second, 1-minute, and 2-minute repetitions in the "Speed Endurance Training" table, will provide a good stimulus.

Muscle Fiber Type

While there's a debate as to whether true muscle fiber conversion occurs (i.e., whether one fiber type transforms into another), there's no denying that muscle fibers can take on the characteristics of other fiber types. Specifically, a conditioning program like the SpeedRunner system can trigger a partial "transformation" of fast-twitch (Type IIx) fibers into intermediate fast-twitch (Type IIa) fibers. Intermediate fibers have more capillaries (small blood vessels) and mitochondria (aerobic-energy producing factories) than fast-twitch fibers. That means they receive more oxygen and create more aerobic energy than fast-twitch fibers. The result is better endurance. The downside is less force production and a slower firing rate than fast-twitch fibers. Wiemann and Tidow suggested this is why the best sprinters *start* with a greater percentage of fast-twitch fibers. Even when some of these fast-twitch fibers transform, enabling better endurance, plenty of others don't, ensuring retention of the power and fast contraction rates that drive top speed. If you start out with fewer fast-twitch fibers, however, don't worry that SpeedRunner training will forever change them into intermediate fibers. When you reduce your training volume and/or intensity, they change back. In fact, by alternating periods of heavy training with periods of limited training, you can manipulate the characteristics of these faster fibers to suit your sport.

Near-Maximal Speed Endurance

Most team-sports athletes don't worry about their extended-sprint times—for 100, 200, or 400 meters. Most sprinters do. But while sprinters must focus on this aspect of speed endurance, many team-sports athletes should, too. If you play a position that might be called upon to stack sprints one on top of another—say, a defensive back who covers a receiver deep, intercepts the ball, and returns it 80 to 90 yards for a score—you'll need extended-sprint endurance. A 2015 study on speed endurance in soccer players found that alternating 20-second all-out efforts with 40 seconds of recovery was highly likely to produce improvement in 200-yard sprint time. The authors suggest, "Shorter rest intervals may limit the [replenishing] of phosphocreatine (CP)... This would in turn tax glycolysis to a greater extent." In other words, a limited recovery period short-circuits your phosphagen system's ability to produce ATP, forcing fast glycolysis to act as your primary energy provider during the first few seconds of the new sprint repetition. As a result, fast glycolysis gets more work, which in turn produces a more effective adaptation.

Repeated-Sprint Endurance

The ability to sustain high velocity for multiple repeated sprints—to sprint, recover, sprint again, recover, sprint, rinse, repeat—is one of the most prized skills for team-sports athletes. Echoing multiple studies, Iaia et al. found that the best way to build repeated-sprint endurance is to mix short sprints with longer recoveries. Soccer players who alternated 20-second sprints with 2-minute recoveries improved significantly in the average speed of each repeated sprint. In contrast, players who alternated 20-second sprints with shorter 40-second recoveries didn't improve (and might have gotten worse). The researchers concluded that developing sustained speed and power requires completing each repetition at goal intensity. That means longer recovery, so that your energy systems have time to restock their shelves (and so that harmful by-products can be eliminated) before beginning your next rep. Players who used the short sprint/long recovery program also improved an average of 10 percent in the Yo-Yo Intermittent Recovery Test, one of the most widely used tests in sports science for measuring speed endurance (see topendsports.com/testing/yo-yo-intermittent-levels.htm for an explanation of the test and youtube.com/watch?v=nkOk_P5VnOA for a video).

Hill Work

Longer hill repeats (or a large volume of short hill sprints) are a good option for speed endurance. You'll work your energy systems just like you would during normal sprinting, but you'll increase the force requirements for your muscle fibers—meaning you'll recruit (and train) more fibers. If you've got hills in your area and aren't overly fatigued from the rest of your training program, you'll want to give this option a shot.

Speed Endurance Training

TRAINING TARGET	WEEK	REPETITIONS	EFFORT	RECOVERY	NOTES
		OPTION 1			
	1	2 × 150 m	95%	250 m walk/jog	If you don't have access to a track, change the reps in this workout to 20 sec. and the recovery to a 2 min. walk/jog.
	2	4 × 150 m	95%	250 m walk/jog	
	3	6 × 150 m	95%	250 m walk/jog	
	4	8 × 150 m	95%	250 m walk/jog	
Repeated Speed Endurance		**OPTION 2**			
	1	Hill Repeats: 2 × 20 sec.	95%	Walk down the hill; wait 2–3 min. total between reps.	Your hill should be steep enough to be challenging, but not so steep that it significantly changes your normal stride.
	2	Hill Repeats: 4 × 20 sec.	95%		
	3	Hill Repeats: 6 × 20 sec.	95%		
	4	Hill Repeats: 6 × 30 sec.	95%		
		OPTION 3			
	1	20 sec. × 4	90–95%	40 sec. jogging	Alternate between running at 90–95% of your top-end speed and jogging; run on a track, trail, or the road.
	2	20 sec. × 6	90–95%	40 sec. jogging	
	3	20 sec. × 8	90–95%	40 sec. jogging	
Near-Maximal Speed Endurance	4	20 sec. × 10	90–95%	40 sec. jogging	
		OPTION 4			
	1	20 sec. × 6	85-90%	40 sec. jogging	Alternate between running at 85–90% of your top-end speed and jogging; run on a track, trail, or the road.
	2	20 sec. × 10	85-90%	40 sec. jogging	
	3	20 sec. × 12-15	85-90%	40 sec. jogging	
	4	20 sec. × 14-20	85-90%	40 sec. jogging	
		OPTION 5			
	1	Distance running: 20-30 min.	65%	---	*For week 4, continue the workout until you can't do another rep, for a maximum of 20 reps.
	2	8 × 1 min.	85-90%	2 min. jogging	
	3	6 × 2 min.	85-90%	2 min. jogging	
Aerobic System	4	30 sec.*	90%	30 sec. jog at 65%	
		OPTION 6			
	1	Distance running: 20-30 min.	65%	---	Distance running is an extra weekly workout that can be performed during the same week as any workout in this table.
	2	Distance running: 20-30 min.	65%	---	
	3	Distance running: 20-30 min.	65%	---	
	4	Distance running: 20-30 min.	65%	---	

Note: Supplement your SpeedRunner training with 1–2 speed endurance workouts per week.

CHAPTER 7 FINAL WORD

Just as different muscle fiber types combine to power every athletic move you make, your three energy systems coordinate to make sure you always have adequate ATP for those moves. If you choose to add extra sessions from the "Speed Endurance Training" table to your regular SpeedRunner training, keep the following guidelines in mind:

1/ Never train speed endurance on the same day as a SpeedRunner session.
2/ The day after maximum velocity training is your best bet.
3/ Choose one option from Options 1 to 5 that suits you and stick with that progression. (Note that Option 6 is only utilized *in addition* to one of these options.)
4/ You can train speed endurance as long as 8 to 12 weeks (you can switch options every 4 weeks, or you can alternate a couple options from week to week, as long as you stick with each option's established progression).
5/ Add easy distance running (Option 6), if desired, any time you want.

Kyle Busch wouldn't line up for the Daytona 500 with a half-tank of gas, and you shouldn't step onto the field, court, or track without your energy systems running at full capacity.

8

RECOVERY AND SUPERCOMPENSATION

Peyton Manning, former quarterback of the NFL's Indianapolis Colts and Denver Broncos, underwent four neck surgeries between February 2010 and September 2011, and he flew to Europe four times to undergo alternative therapies, including electro-stimulation and a controversial stem cell procedure. It was all an attempt to reverse nerve damage and resultant muscle atrophy. At one point, according to Sally Jenkins in a 2013 profile of Manning, the perennial league MVP tried to throw a ball 10 yards to his friend, Todd Helton, only to have it nose-dive after 5 yards. Accused of joking around by Helton, Manning said, "Man, I wish I was." Manning lost his entire 2011 season to rehab. For three months, he wasn't allowed to touch a football. After that, he spent weeks facing a mirror and practicing his throwing move. Finally, he went to work with David Cutcliffe, his former offensive coordinator at the University of

>> **RECOVERY**

An interval of inactivity or reduced exercise between workout repetitions; repairing muscle and connective tissue damage plus restocking energy systems and neurotransmitters post-workout; a return to baseline fitness

Tennessee (Manning's alma mater), and relearned the basics: how to grip the ball, his setup, his release. With weakened triceps muscles from the nerve damage, Manning compensated by training his legs, core, and other arm muscles to be their strongest.

The Colts, not convinced that rehab had done the trick, released Manning. Denver signed him in March 2012, but four months later, Peyton's father, Archie, a former NFL quarterback himself, told Jenkins that Manning's form was still iffy. "Wasn't bad, wasn't ugly," he said, "but it wasn't Peyton." Manning persevered. And started to look good. And then better than good—*great*. During the 2012 season, he threw for 37 touchdowns and 4,659 yards, earning his 12th trip to the Pro Bowl (the NFL's all-star game). The next season, he set NFL records with 55 touchdown passes and 5,477 yards, earning his 5th MVP award and a trip to the Super Bowl. The Broncos lost that game, but two years later, with Manning still at the helm, they won it. And Manning completed one of the greatest comebacks—recovering from what could have been career-ending surgeries—in sports history.

No one's asking you to pull a Peyton Manning.

All you need to do is recover from one repetition to the next, and then from workout to workout. This means practicing patience, and allowing your body to do what it does best—assess damage, repair, and rebuild stronger than before.

WHAT'S RECOVERY?

RECOVERY ISN'T A SINGLE, SPECIFIC ITEM on your training to-do list. Instead, it's a wide-ranging action plan that guides your effort level and fatigue during workouts, returns you to baseline fitness post-workout, and then rebuilds your body to be stronger than it was pre-training.

Outside of a few temporary nervous system adaptations, you don't get faster, stronger, or quicker while you train. Those things happen while you're recovering. That's when new nervous system pathways get hardwired. That's when your muscles and connective tissue get repaired. That's when neurotransmitters and hormones get replaced, your energy systems get restocked, and your hydration levels get filled back to the brim. Then, and only then, something magical happens: Your body, seeking to shield itself against a future training challenge like the one it just faced, rebuilds a little bit stronger than it was pre-training.

Recovery Strategies

The table below shows recovery strategies used by athletes, coaches, and health professionals to aid recovery before, during, and after a workout. "Harmful" activities, which negatively impact your training, performance, or health, are marked with a skull and crossbones (multiple skulls and crossbones means *more* harmful). "Ineffective" strategies neither hurt nor help you. They might even make you feel good, which can be a positive in and of itself, but they won't boost your 40 time. "Effective" and "Highly Effective" strategies should be part of your routine.

STRATEGY	Harmful	Ineffective	Effective	Highly effective
Active recovery days				✔
Alcohol	☠☠			
Anti-inflammatories (acute injury)			✔	
Anti-inflammatories (muscle soreness—age 40+)			✔	
Anti-inflammatories (muscle soreness)	☠☠			
Antioxidants	☠			
Chiropractic solutions		✔		
Cold water immersion	☠			
Compression gear		✔		
Days off (due to fatigue)			✔	
Diet			✔	
Foam rolling		✔		
Heat therapy			✔	
Ice (acute injury)			✔	
Ice (muscle soreness)	☠			
Just relax				✔
Kinesio tape		✔		
Massage		✔		
Performance-Enhancing Drugs	☠☠☠			
Post-workout carbs				✔
Protein (post-workout & pre-bedtime)			✔	
Recovery interval manipulation				✔
Rehydration				✔
Sleep				✔
Static stretching (post-workout)			✔	
Static stretching (pre-workout)	☠☠			
Vitamin supplements		✔		
Whole-body strengthening				✔

Training is planting seeds. Recovery is when your crops grow. In this chapter, we'll look at a few different aspects of recovery:

▸ **Hard/Easy:** You can't train hard every day and expect to recover (or improve).
▸ **Supercompensation:** This is the ultimate goal of recovery between hard workouts.
▸ **Overtraining:** The arch enemy of proper recovery that must be avoided.
▸ **Beneficial recovery practices:** From active recovery days to protein supplementation, these practices should be a part of your program.
▸ **Harmful or ineffective recovery practices:** Whether harmful or simply useless as recovery tools, these are practices to avoid.

Some athletes have a hard time making room for recovery in their program. They would rather train hard for every minute of every workout. That's a recipe for fatigue, reduced fitness, and injury—and for losing to athletes who embrace recovery to become better athletes.

LET'S TALK RECOVERY

IT'S NOT THE TRAINING YOU DO THAT COUNTS. It's the training your body can recover from.

Your body is capable of only incremental improvement from one hard workout to the next. There's no value in putting yourself through a brutal workout from which your body can't recover—or through a string of workouts that continuously breaks you down. You don't get faster. You don't get stronger or quicker. You don't get any fitter. You simply get tired. And maybe burned out, overtrained, or injured. Let's go through some of the basics of recovery and anti-recovery.

Hard/Easy and Supercompensation

Hard/easy is the most basic rule of training. If you train hard one day, you take the next day easy. "Easy" is not a synonym for "off." Vern Gambetta, whose resume includes stints as director of USA Track & Field coaching education and conditioning coach and consultant for professional teams in the NFL, NBA, NHL, MLB, and soccer—and who is the author of several books and more than 100 articles on sports performance and coaching—has identified four steps for recovery and supercompensation, which we'll summarize here.

Training Stress: You train, and your body gets fatigued, accompanied by some muscle and connective tissue damage, and by energy system and neurotransmitter depletion. As a result, you are *less capable* of performing than before you started the workout.

Recovery: Lighter training or inactivity allows energy stores and performance to return to baseline (i.e., the same fitness you possessed before doing the workout in step one).

Supercompensation: You get better than you were before. "This is the adaptive rebound above the baseline," writes Gambetta. "It is described as a rebound response because the body is essentially rebounding from the low point of greatest fatigue. This supercompensation effect is not only a physiological response but also a psychological and technical response."

Decline: At the peak of supercompensation, you either apply an increased training stimulus—and temporarily regress, due to a new round of fatigue, muscle damage, energy system depletion, etc.—or you fail to apply the stimulus, in which case you begin to lose the beneficial adaptations of supercompensation (a process called "detraining").

As a coach, one of the most frequent complaints I hear from athletes about scheduled recovery is this: "But I feel good!" Look, you're supposed to feel good after recovery. You've healed. Your energy systems are topped off. But that's not a green light to train hard. First, you must wait for supercompensation to occur. If you're unwilling to wait for improvement, then what's the point?

> **》 SUPERCOMPENSATION**
>
> Your body's improvement post-workout; wherein training weakens you, recovery returns you to baseline fitness, and supercompensation leaves you stronger than pre-training

DOMS

DOMS (delayed onset muscles soreness) is muscular pain experienced by athletes in the aftermath of excessive exercise. You'll start to feel DOMS by the day after your workout, but its symptoms won't peak for 48 to 72 hours. While it's tempting to use heat or cold treatments to temporarily relieve pain and recover some performance capacity, the reality is that you'll need to take a couple easy days—or, better yet, a couple days off. Symptoms should be gone within a week. Consider DOMS a warning: Train too hard, get injured.

Overtraining

I once asked Dr. Jack Daniels, named "The World's Best Coach" by *Runner's World* magazine, for his advice on overtraining syndrome. His answer was two words long: "Avoid it." And, really, that's what you need to know in a nutshell. Overtraining is what it sounds like: It's training too hard, too long, and too often. If a workout is way too hard, what I call a "monster workout," then "too long" can be that single workout. When overtraining hits, you'll find that exercise that once seemed easy is no longer possible. Symptoms include impaired performance, heavy legs, muscle and joint pain, lethargy, insomnia, clumsiness, weight loss, elevated heart rate, and increased thirst at night. And here's the kicker: Once overtraining strikes, it takes weeks or months of limited activity—or inactivity—to recover from it. If you start feeling symptoms, cut back on your training immediately. If you practice proper recovery strategies, you'll probably never have to worry about this syndrome.

>> **ACTIVE RECOVERY**
Lighter training post-exercise (i.e., a warm-down) or between hard exercise sessions (i.e., an easy day) to improve and accelerate recovery

LET'S TALK RECOVERY PRACTICES

THERE'S NO BETTER RECOVERY PRACTICE than smart, patient training that targets incremental improvement and long-term goals. Still, there are additional strategies you can employ. Some work, some don't, and some will even rob you of the improvement you've worked so hard to acquire.

Beneficial Practices

ACTIVE RECOVERY

There's debate in the exercise-science community over the value of the warm-down (e.g., easy jogging or exercises post-training or competition). But there's no debate within the athletes' community. It works. "Continued blood flow to the skeletal muscle bed," writes Lance C. Dalleck in a 2016 article for the American Council on Exercise (ACE), "promotes the resynthesis of CrP [creatine phosphate] and glycogen stores. It also facilitates the removal of [acidic] protons." In other words, active recovery allows you to quickly restock energy supplies, and it limits fatigue. But active recovery doesn't end with your warm-down. During the session(s) that follows a hard workout, you should limit the volume and/or intensity of exercise. This allows reinforcement of the hard workout's ongoing adaptations without short-circuiting the process by adding a new, heavy training load. Active recovery periods are great for practicing individual skills, teamwork, and other aspects of your sport that don't require an all-out effort.

DIET

This isn't a diet or nutrition book. So consider this entry merely a reminder that you need a good diet to compete. It's also a reminder that most of the calories you burn during intense exercise come from carbohydrates—so eat plenty of them. Eat plenty of high-quality proteins and fats, too. And stay away from diet sodas and sugar—they're fitness killers.

HEAT

Do not use heat for an acute injury. At least not for the first 24 hours post-injury, as you'll increase swelling, pain, joint immobility, and recovery time. After two or three days, however, heat can help speed recovery by bringing blood flow to the injured area. If you're stiff from a previous workout, heat applied pre-exercise will help loosen muscles and connective tissue. A 2013 study on tendon flexibility found that applying heat to your knee can reduce the force required to move the joint by 25 percent. Heat can be applied with pads (e.g., hydrocollator packs), a water bottle, and the like. Post-workout, a warm bath might be a good bet. A 2015 study had participants spend 40 minutes immersed in a warm bath (40° C, 104° F) to see if it would trigger adaptations usually associated with heat-acclimatization (i.e., training in the heat). Researchers found that six days of a warm-bath regimen lowered core temperature during both rest and exercise, initiated sweating at lower temperatures, reduced perceived exertion, and improved 5K times run in the heat (33° C, 91.4° F) by 4.9 percent—moreover, the authors contend that the improvements would hold for both temperate and hot environments. Be sensible if you go this route. Once you have the adaptations, turn down the heat.

JUST RELAX

Many of the athletes I've coached initially approached me because they'd been chronically injured and heard I specialize in getting athletes back on their feet. Invariably, these athletes had been using multiple rehab strategies for their injuries: ice, heat, anti-inflammatories, PT-prescribed exercises, chiropractic adjustments, orthotics . . . you name it. One athlete ran with magnets on her feet. Another slept with a painful, lower-leg night splint. The first thing I tell these athletes is this: "Stop everything you're doing." It's like picking at a scab, this hyper-focus on one small, injured area of the body. If the injury wasn't already there, the extra poking, rubbing, heating, cooling, taping, stressing, and whatnot would likely cause an injury. Your body is a biomechanical miracle. Sometimes, you just gotta let it recover on its own. You'd be amazed at its ability to regenerate. Yes, there are good rehab exercises and recovery strategies. But, no, they aren't improved by wearing magnet-enhanced knee straps.

POST-TRAINING SNACKS AND REHYDRATION

If you want to feel better for tomorrow's workout, then consume a carbohydrate snack immediately after today's workout (within the first 15 to 30 minutes). Consume a second carbohydrate snack 60 minutes later. During this post-workout period, your body restocks muscle glycogen (carbs) at an accelerated rate. So plan on 50 to 100 grams of carbs—twice—to take advantage. Also, the faster you rehydrate, the faster your body will return to baseline. Drink water immediately after practice or competition, then continue drinking until your needle's on "full." If you utilize a sports drink, switch to water once you've ingested enough carbs and/or protein.

PROTEIN

Both scientific and anecdotal evidence show that protein supplementation improves recovery from training and competition. As coach Steve Magness told me in an interview for my first book, *Build Your Running Body*, "If you regularly take in a spike of 15 grams of protein, you'll get a spike in muscle protein synthesis." That spike leads to quicker muscle repair, increased strength, and gains in aerobic and anaerobic strength. In addition to 4 or 5 spikes of 15 to 20 grams during the day, a spike of 30 grams at bedtime promotes accelerated muscle repair while you sleep.

RECOVERY INTERVAL MANIPULATION

Too many athletes believe that the proper recovery interval between repetitions is the shortest one. It's not. The correct recovery interval is the one that focuses the training stimulus on the muscle fiber types and energy systems you're targeting. Although it may sound counterintuitive, longer recoveries put the emphasis on faster-acting energy systems, while shorter recoveries favor slower-acting energy systems. For example, if you run 20-second repetitions at 95 percent effort, this is how the recovery interval affects your targeted energy system.

> ▸ **2-minute recovery interval:** Longer recovery allows your phosphagen system to replenish its creatine phosphate stores. That makes this system a strong first responder for your next repetition—and ensures that your fastest fibers, which produce the most force, will have adequate energy to drive that rep. Your body will also limit fast glycolysis with each subsequent repetition, further focusing the workout on your phosphagen system.

> ▸ **40-second recovery interval:** Since the phosphagen system doesn't have time to fully replenish its CP, each subsequent repetition relies more on fast glycolysis.

> ▸ **20-second recovery interval:** Since neither the phosphagen system nor fast glycolysis has time to recover, each subsequent repetition relies more on your aerobic system.

The specifics of the above example work only for 20-second repetitions at 95 percent effort. When you change the length and/or intensity of a repetition, the recovery interval required to target specific muscle fiber types and energy systems changes, too. So trust the recommended recovery intervals for exercises and drills in this book (and for those given to you by your coaches). It's not about training hard and feeling the burn. It's about training smart and getting better.

SLEEP

Extra sleep is a proven recovery tool. In a 2008 study, swimmers from Stanford University men's and women's teams slept 10 hours a day for 6 to 7 weeks. The result was an average 0.51-second improvement in a 15-yard swim, a 0.15-second improvement in reaction time, and a 0.1-second improvement in turn time. A 2011 study extended the experiment to members of Stanford's basketball team. After 5 to 7 weeks of 10 hours of sleep per day, the players improved their average times for a 282-foot sprint (baseline to half-court, back to baseline, then to full-court, then back to baseline) from 16.2 to 15.5 seconds, improved free throw accuracy by 9 percent, and improved 3-point field goal accuracy by 9.2 percent. Cheri Mah, the lead author of the two studies, has also worked with Stanford's teams for football, tennis, golf, cross country, and track. She concluded that "athletes across all sports can greatly benefit from extra sleep and gain the additional competitive edge to perform at their highest level."

WHOLE-BODY STRENGTHENING

Discussing the ability of pro athletes to recover quickly from injury, sports medicine expert John Xerogeanes, M.D., said in a 2015 interview, "Biology only lets you recover so fast, so it's not like pro athletes' cells are going to heal faster than our cells. But the other structures around their knees—or whatever they've hurt—are so strong and so much better than ours, they're going to protect the part that's healing and help it get stronger in less time." Those structures are "strong" and "better than ours" because pro athletes train them to be that way. Whole-body strengthening, like that included in the SpeedRunner system, gives you the same edge as the pros.

Recovery No-No's

ALCOHOL

A 2013 study on alcohol and testosterone production had men drink an average of 1.09 grams of alcohol per kilogram of body weight immediately after strenuous weight lifting. For a 150-pound man, that's about 5.3 drinks. The result was that men's testosterone levels rose an average of 78 percent. While higher testosterone would normally be considered a desired result post-workout, researchers cautioned that testosterone increased because alcohol destroyed the muscle cells' testosterone receptors—in other words, there was more testosterone in the bloodstream because muscles could no longer use it. Other studies suggest that alcohol damages the cells that produce testosterone and inhibits recovery and muscle adaptations. And studies clearly document lower testosterone levels in heavy drinkers. Bottom line? While a couple drinks a day might not hurt you, they definitely won't help you.

ANTI-INFLAMMATORIES

In their book, *The Runner's Body*, Ross Tucker and Jonathan Dugas explain that inflammation, far from being an impediment to recovery and improved performance, triggers specialized cells (neutrophils, macrophages, and monocytes) to clear away damaged muscle tissue, paving the way for the creation of stronger, more durable muscle fibers. Interrupting this process derails your body's ability to recover and adapt. "For most people, with normal training, you probably don't need to do anything about inflammation," says Dugas, in a 2010 interview. "Even during hard training, you don't need to do anything except follow the standard training process of built-in rest periods." One exception: Masters athletes have been shown to achieve greater strength gains while using anti-inflammatories (and acetaminophen). Still, the risks associated with serial use of these drugs (including kidney, heart, and bone damage) make this a poor recovery strategy.

ANTIOXIDANTS

Antioxidants (vitamins C, A, and E are examples) reduce cell damage from free radicals (harmful molecules that can form during exercise). But here's the thing: You need some of that damage to stimulate training adaptations. Take away oxidative stress, and you simply won't get the same performance boost. Studies have shown antioxidants having no effect on mitochondrial gains (i.e., increased aerobic energy production), with some studies even showing negative effects. Your best strategy is to eat fruits and vegetables, which are naturally high in antioxidants, and skip the exorbitant volume of antioxidants found in many multivitamins and supplements.

CHIROPRACTIC SOLUTIONS

Daniel David Palmer invented the field of chiropractics in 1897. Palmer taught that misalignment of your bones, mainly your spine (called "vertebral subluxations"), is the underlying cause of all disease. Despite this pseudoscientific heritage, I sent my athletes to chiropractors for treatment of sciatica and lower back spasms for almost

30 years. Some athletes reported relief. Others did not. Finally, I stopped endorsing this route. There is simply no evidence to recommend chiropractic over placebo treatment. A 2012 review of 20 chiropractic trials, including 2,674 participants, concluded that chiropractic spinal manipulative therapy was "no more effective in participants with acute low-back pain" than sham treatments and placebos. And science writer Paul Ingraham, in his 2016 update to his article, "Does Chiropractic Work?," notes that "if SMT [spinal manipulative therapy] works, it shouldn't be taking over a century to prove it." Like many ineffective recovery strategies, the fact that most people feel good after chiropractic work doesn't mean that it's triggering a beneficial physiological effect.

COLD WATER IMMERSION AND ICING

Years ago, I'd finish every workout with 15 to 20 minutes in an ice-water bath, which I believed would reduce inflammation and ward off injury. The only problem: I was constantly injured. A 2015 investigation may explain why. "Cold water immersion attenuated [reduced] long-term gains in muscle and strength," the study found. "It also blunted the activation of key proteins and satellite cells in skeletal muscle up to two days after strength exercise." Dr. Jonathan Peake, one of the study's authors, cautioned that athletes who include strength training in their programs "should reconsider using cold-water immersion as a recovery aid." As with anti-inflammatories and antioxidants, this strategy disrupts the normal process of recovery. That said, if you suffer an acute injury, both cold-water immersion and ice can help limit swelling. Also, if you're simply trying to reduce soreness for a specific practice or competition, cold therapy can do the trick—just don't make it a long-term practice.

HIGH-TECH REHABILITATION

"The media talks about stem cells, PRP injections, cool rehab machines," says Dr. Xerogeanes, "but [they're expensive] and honestly, they're all unproven anyway. You hear about antigravity treadmills, but you can get the same benefits running underwater in a pool." None of these high-tech recovery therapies are technically "no-no's." Instead, they're pricey and unproven. A 2013 review of six studies on platelet rich plasma (PRP) injections found that they "may have beneficial effects" in cases of moderate knee damage, but it also found they increased the risk of adverse events—in other words, *the small benefit might not outweigh the risk*. A 2017 Australian meta-analysis of 18 studies concluded that there "is good evidence to support the use of a single injection of LR-PRP [leukocyte-rich PRP] under ultrasound guidance in tendinopathy."

Tendinopathy refers to conditions that cause tendon pain. But *PT in Motion*, the official magazine of the American Physical Therapy Association, reports that some of this study's "details remain fuzzy." Honestly, not only are other recovery practices mentioned in this book proven to be effective, they're also cheaper.

KINESIO TAPE

The maker of Kinesio Tape (KT) boasts that it "alleviates discomfort and facilitates lymphatic drainage by microscopically lifting the skin." But a 2014 review of 12 trials involving 495 participants, published in the *Journal of Physiotherapy*, concluded that "Kinesio Taping was no better than sham taping/placebo and active comparison groups [i.e., groups that performed basic exercises]." A 2012 review of studies likewise found "insufficient evidence to support the use of KT following musculoskeletal injury"—although it did suggest that there might be a short-term "perceived" benefit (i.e., you feel good wearing it, so you assume you're getting some benefit).

PEDS (PERFORMANCE-ENHANCING DRUGS)

In the 2006 Tour de France, Floyd Landis "recovered" from a disastrous Stage 16 to perform a 75-mile solo breakaway in Stage 17. He won the stage by almost six minutes, then three days later claimed the overall Tour de France championship. Less than one month later, he was disqualified for having ridden Stage 17 with 11 times the normal amount of testosterone in his system. He'd cheated. Landis isn't alone. Of the all-time top-10 male 100-meter sprinters, 8 have either been banned for PED use or associated with it. And PED scandals have damaged the credibility of almost every major sport. But PED users aren't just cheaters and frauds. They're also putting their health, even their lives, at risk. In the years since synthetic EPO was introduced in 1989, more than 100 international bike racers have died in their sleep or dropped dead from heart attacks—known risks of EPO abuse. And steroid and HGH use has been linked to shrunken testicles, weakened tendons, liver damage, high blood pressure, increased risk of heart disease, and much more. Yes, PEDs will allow you to recover more quickly—and with far greater supercompensation—but at what price?

STATIC STRETCHING, MASSAGE, AND COMPRESSION GEAR

Stretching, massage, and compression gear are popular with athletes. But are they helpful? "Results from numerous review articles show no beneficial effect toward post-exercise recovery from either stretching, massage, or compression garments," writes Dalleck in his summary of recovery for ACE. He adds, however, that some people do feel better when using these strategies. He also notes that no adverse effects are associated with any of them. As an athlete and coach, let me add an experience-based caveat to Dalleck's conclusion. Pre-workout static stretching doesn't help performance (studies show it does the opposite) and increases the risk of injury for those who are new to stretching. Post-workout static stretching, on the other hand, will leave you less stiff for the next day's training. Also, some forms of dynamic stretching—active isolated stretching (AIS) and proprioceptive neuromuscular facilitation stretching (PNF)—will improve your muscles' range of motion.

VITAMINS AND OTHER SUPPLEMENTS

We've discussed the danger of overdoing antioxidants, but what about other supplements? Beyond protein, which we already gave a thumbs-up, the news isn't good. Peer-reviewed studies rarely confirm what supplement manufacturers claim. The truth is that your need for supplements generally arises from the fact that processing removes nutrients from the foods you find at the supermarket. My advice is to buy real food—food that hasn't had its nutrients stripped—and avoid supplements, which don't provide the full array of nutrients, vitamins, minerals, herbs, enzymes, and so on that are found in natural foodstuffs. That said, there is *one* supplement that I recommend wholeheartedly—a supplement that has been proven to fight cancer, lower cholesterol, shed unwanted pounds, build muscle, improve nervous system function, extend lifespan, and keep your bones strong. That supplement is this: smart training. And that's the supplement that SpeedRunner offers.

CHAPTER 8 FINAL WORD

Recovery is improvement. There are beneficial and harmful practices that can affect your recovery, but your main focus should be on performing the correct volume of training at the correct intensity, and then implementing a period of lighter training and rest while your body repairs and rebuilds—after which you'll begin the cycle again, repeating it over and over until you achieve your peak performance.

9

SPEEDRUNNER WORKOUTS

The SpeedRunner exercises and drills are presented in five sections:

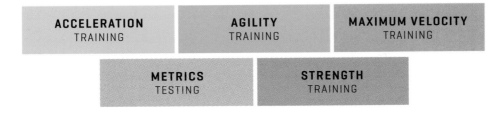

Each section contains exercises and drills specifically related to the section topic. Entries for each exercise and drill include:

▸ An introduction to the exercise or drill
▸ Workout volume (e.g., number of reps and sets)
▸ Step-by-step text instruction
▸ Illustrative photos
▸ Additional tips as needed
▸ A course setup diagram with instructions on cone layout (where applicable)

Choose a SpeedRunner schedule from Chapter 10 or create your own program. If you follow one of the schedules, be aware that the number of sets and reps might not match those prescribed for exercises in this chapter. There are two reasons why:

1/ The schedules incorporate incremental training principles (that is, you start with less volume and intensity for exercises, then build both from session to session, and from week to week).

2/ Within each session, the schedules meticulously balance the workload delivered to your muscles and nervous system while also focusing on energy-system conservation and recovery. This sometimes requires altering the prescribed sets and repetitions you'd use for an exercise were you to perform it separately from a session.

If you choose to create your own program, you'll find all the information you need to make informed decisions in the book's previous chapters.

A NOTE ON VOLUME AND RECOVERY

MOST OF THE EXERCISES AND DRILLS offer a range for volume. For example, 3-Bounce & Run recommends 2–3 reps of 15–20 yards. Choose the volume that best represents your current fitness. New to training? Opt for the lower end when it comes to volume. If you're sharpening skills and fitness developed over the course of years, you may want to begin with more volume. Either way, your fitness will improve, and you'll soon be mastering more challenging workouts.

For recovery between sets, reps, and exercises, use this rule of thumb:

▸ 1–3 minutes of recovery following sets and single-rep exercises (e.g., a hill sprint)
▸ 10–30 seconds (or however long it takes you to switch exercises) during circuit training

That said, if you need more recovery time, take it. Remember, it's not the training you do that counts; it's the training from which your body can recover. If you overdo it, you won't get faster; you'll get injured, sick, or burned out.

ACCELERATION TRAINING

WALK/JOGGING

The simplest way to warm up for training that involves running is walk/jogging. That's because you literally warm up. When you walk and jog, your muscles produce aerobic energy, but you only capture about 25 percent of that energy for muscle contractions. The rest is lost as body heat—heat that warms your muscles, making them less stiff. When your muscles are limber and your legs feel light, you're ready for action.

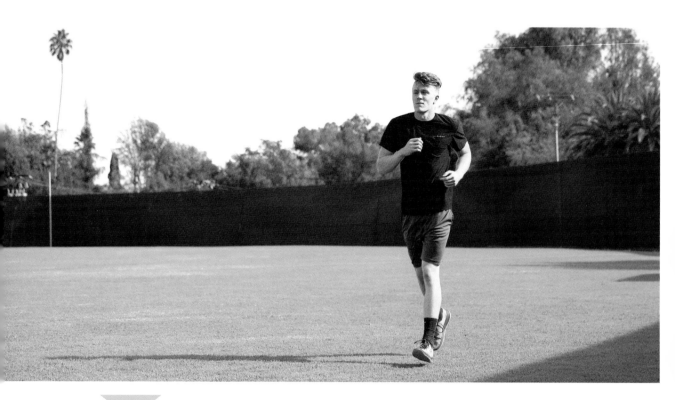

WORKOUT   Walk for a prescribed time and then jog

▸ Begin with easy walking for 1–5 minutes.

▸ Jog at 55–65% effort for 10–12 minutes (15–18 minutes for athletes age 40+).

COACH'S 2 CENTS

Some athletes think walking is a waste of time. Good athletes know better. Injuries often occur during the first few minutes of training—muscles that aren't warm lack flexibility and force-production capacity. Walking warms up your muscles so that you can safely transition to jogging and then to intense exercise. **Note: This is not an acceleration exercise; it's a warm-up exercise to be used prior to SpeedRunner sessions.**

BUILDUPS 4-2-2

This exercise is a great warm-up for those who find strides more engaging than jogging. Also, a 4-2-2 buildup better prepares an athlete's nervous system for the workout intensity of a SpeedRunner session. Mixing strides of increasing intensity with walking raises body temperature, reduces muscle stiffness, and prepares the nervous system for the faster work ahead.

123

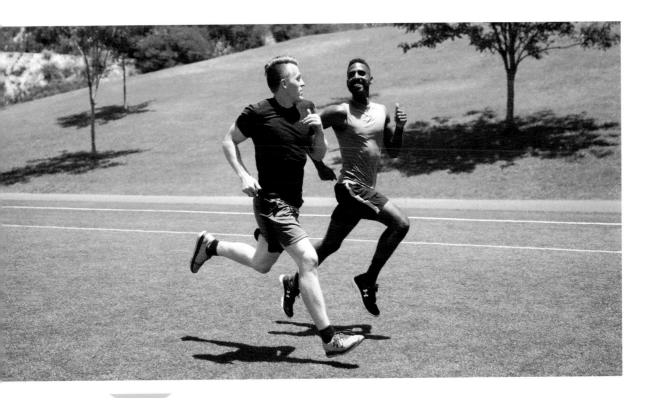

WORKOUT **1 set of all strides and walk periods**

▶ Begin with 4 strides of 60–100 yards, at 50–65% of maximum effort. Walk back to the start line after each stride.

▶ Run 2 more strides, same length, at 65–75% of maximum effort. Again, walk back to the start line after each stride.

▶ Finish with 2 strides, same length, at 75–85% of maximum effort. Walk back to the start line after each stride.

COACH'S 2 CENTS

Don't overdo the effort on these strides; this is only a warm-up. If you're approaching 90% maximum effort, that's a workout, not a warm-up.

3-BOUNCE & RUN

This exercise prepares you for game-time acceleration. Few sports allow you the luxury of starting your sprint from statue-like stillness, so it's important that you train your nervous system to initiate a powerful start when you're already on the move.

124

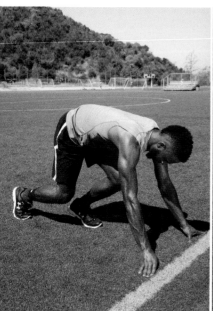 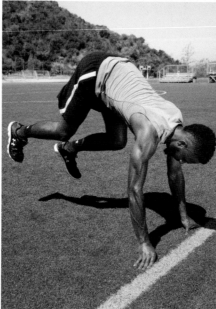 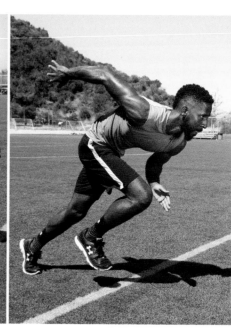

WORKOUT **2–3 reps of 15–20 yards**

▸ Start from a 4-point stance (see box).

▸ Bounce 3 times off the balls of your feet, lifting both legs at the same time. As you land the third time, explode into a sprint.

COACH'S 2 CENTS

Bouncing three times from a set position pre-tunes your muscles for action. Also, although you'll extend your arms in a 4-point stance, take care not to lock out your elbows.

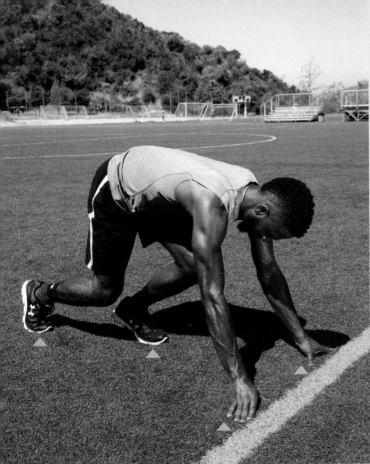

4-POINT STANCE

(4 "points" because you have both feet and both hands on the ground)

▶ Place your left foot about 2 foot-lengths behind the start line, with your right foot another foot back, and take a knee with your right leg.

▶ Place your hands on the start line, slightly wider than shoulder width. Your fingers should point out, thumbs in, forming a bridge.

▶ Push up with your legs until your left knee is bent at 90° and your right knee is at 100°–120°.

▶ Your shoulders should be directly over your hands, arms straight.

▶ Reverse foot placement if your left leg is dominant.

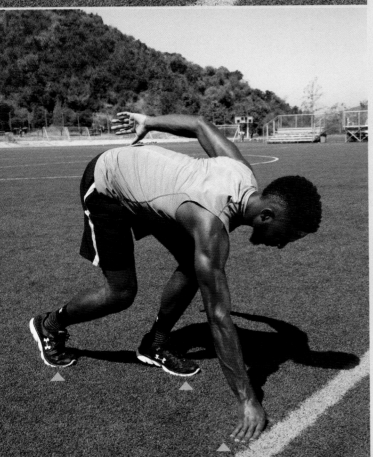

3-POINT STANCE

(3 "points" because you have both feet and one hand on the ground)

▶ Place your left foot about 1–2 foot-lengths behind the start line.

▶ Take a knee with your right leg, positioning that knee parallel to the ball of your left foot, with no more than 6 inches between them.

▶ Place your right hand directly behind the start line, with your fingers pointing out, your thumbs in, forming a bridge.

▶ Push up with your legs until your left knee is bent at 90° and your right knee is at 100–120°.

▶ Your right arm should be straight, with no bend at the elbow.

▶ Extend your left arm behind you, slightly above hip level.

▶ Reverse foot placement if your left leg is dominant.

3-POINT STANCE & SPRINT

A 3-point stance is the start position for many drills, including NFL combine tests such as the 40-yard dash, 20-yard shuttle, and 3-cone drill. You'll use intense concentric contractions (and a triple extension of hip, knee, and ankle) to explode off the start line, and you'll practice the forward body lean that's essential for first-steps acceleration.

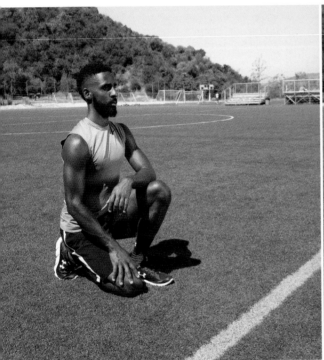
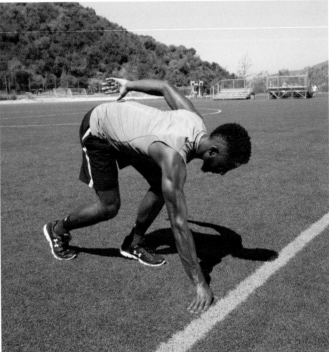

WORKOUT   2–3 reps of 10–20 yards

▸ Begin in a 3-point stance (see p. 125).

▸ On command (external or internal), drive forward for 10–20 yards.

COACH'S 2 CENTS

Rest most of your weight on your legs for better balance and a more explosive start. **Note: Reverse left-right instructions if your left leg is dominant.**

BOUNDING

Bounding is a terrific training drill for both acceleration and maximum velocity. Research has found that it is the only exercise that simulates the EMG model (muscle activation sequence) of actual sprinting, mimicking sprinting's short contact time, large generation of horizontal force, and high-power output. If you could only do one drill, this would be it!

127

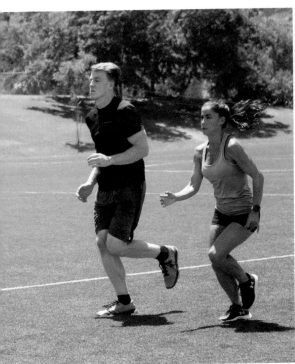
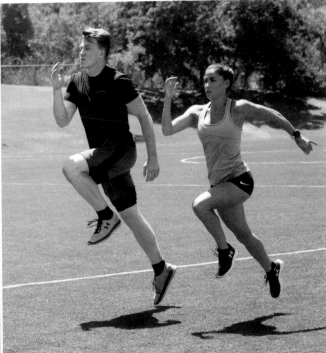

▼ **WORKOUT   1 rep of 20–60 yards**

▸ Build into the drill with a few short hops from one foot to the other.

▸ Drive forward off the ball of one foot, completely extending your push-off leg as you leap forward and up (like Superman taking flight). Hold the position, keeping your front knee raised high for a moment of hang time.

▸ Land on your opposite foot, absorb the impact force, and then quickly spring into another bound. Switch your landing foot with each bound (i.e., this isn't skipping).

COACH'S 2 CENTS

Go for your best combination of distance and height. Although this is an acceleration exercise, it's usually performed as part of a series of maximum velocity technique drills.

JUMP & SPRINT

This exercise uses a standing forward jump to pre-tune your lower limbs and core muscles for the powerful concentric contractions that drive acceleration. As you land the jump, you create stretch-shortening cycles (triggered by eccentric contractions) in your hamstrings, glutes, and calves. Your nervous system harnesses this extra energy to create an explosive start.

128

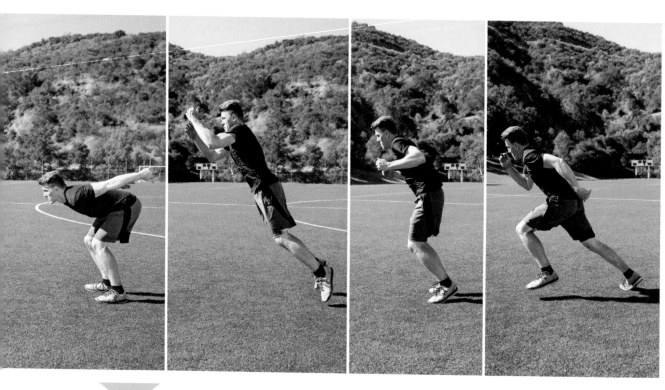

WORKOUT 2–3 reps of 1 jump + 10–15 yards

▶ From a standing position, feet hip-width apart, bend your knees into a squat while drawing both arms behind you.

▶ Jump forward off both feet.

▶ As soon as you land, sprint forward.

COACH'S 2 CENTS

This exercise is especially useful for team-sports athletes who don't regularly utilize a crouched start (e.g., soccer and lacrosse athletes).

RESISTED RUN

Adding resistance through use of a tether allows you to mimic the forward lean of acceleration while working at less than 100 percent effort. When you're sprinting, acceleration lasts 3–5 seconds. With resisted running, you can maintain an acceleration posture for twice as long. You'll develop both strength and horizontal force capacity.

129

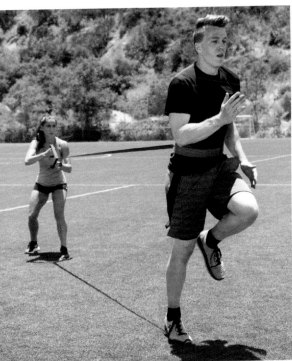
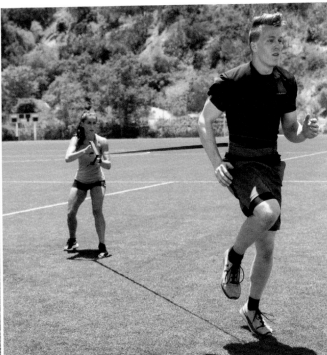

WORKOUT   **2 reps of 5–10 seconds**

▶ Begin from a standing position with your left (or strongest) foot forward and a slight forward lean. The tether should be taut between your harness and your anchor (i.e., a stable object or a person holding the tether).

▶ Sprint at 90–95% effort.

▶ Gradually adopt a forward lean that mimics the period of acceleration you're targeting.

▶ Run in place for 5–10 seconds, maintaining good acceleration form.

COACH'S 2 CENTS

Waist harnesses allow you to apply force in a natural way; shoulder harnesses apply a restraining force too high on your torso. Also, be like Goldilocks when finding your forward lean—not too much, not too little, just riiiiight! While it's easiest to work with a partner, you can also secure the tether to a stable object.

HILL SPRINTS AND STADIUM STEPS

Hill Sprints allow runners to use area topography to recreate the body mechanics used for initial acceleration. Sprinting up a hill replicates acceleration's forward lean. You also use an increased push to drive yourself upward against gravity, building power and horizontal force capacity. If your area lacks hills, stadium steps at your local high school or college offer a similar benefit.

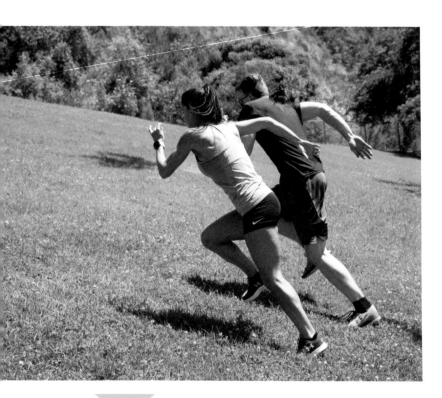

WORKOUT   2–8 reps lasting 8–12 seconds

▸ Choose an appropriately steep hill (see Coach's 2 Cents).

▸ Jog into the sprint for 5–10 yards.

▸ Sprint at 90–95% maximum effort.

COACH'S 2 CENTS

Your hill should be steep, but not so steep that you can't maintain a rough approximation of your normal stride. Also, resist the urge to sprint longer than prescribed—longer is not better. This exercise is fueled by your phosphagen system, which has a max output of 10–15 seconds.

Additional instruction for
STADIUM STEPS

▸ Use 2–3 steps to build up to 90–95% effort.

▸ Climb two steps at a time, pumping your knees while mimicking the intensity you'd use during a hill sprint.

▸ Use the same time-volume prescribed for hill sprints.

Additional instruction for
DOWNHILL SPRINTS

Downhill Sprints increase the load on your quadriceps muscle and improve stride length. Add a longer ground contact time, and this exercise creates a stimulus similar to the Weight Sled Run.

▸ Using the same hill as for Hill Sprints, spend 10–20 yards jogging into the downhill sprint.

▸ Sprint at 85–95% maximum effort for 8–12 seconds. Focus on maintaining form.

MEDBALL PUSH & SPRINT

You'll start by building force with your legs, then with your torso, and finally with your shoulders, chest, and arms. This movement culminates with a push, as you thrust the medball forward as far as you can. Once the medball is released, transition to a sprint, allowing your neuromuscular system to harness the momentum you've created and ignite an explosive start.

131

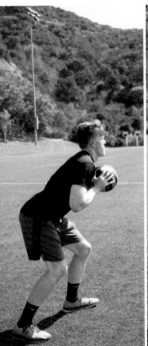
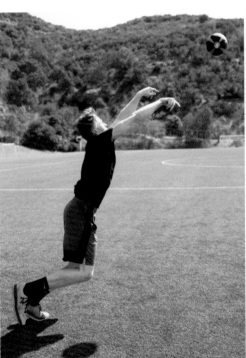
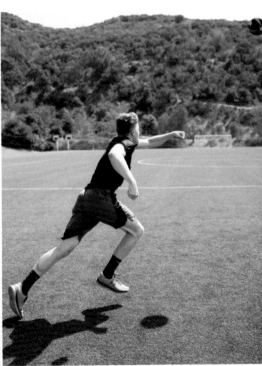

WORKOUT   **2–3 reps of 1 medball push + 10–15 yards**

▸ Begin from a standing position with your left foot (or right foot, if it's your strongest foot) forward, the toes of your right foot even with your left heel, and a slight forward lean.

▸ Hold a medball close to your body, at chest level, with both hands.

▸ Quickly bend at the knees, then explode up while simultaneously propelling the medball forward.

▸ As soon as the medball is out of your hands, sprint forward.

COACH'S 2 CENTS

This exercise is especially useful for athletes who must regularly transition from full-body action to acceleration (e.g., a baseball player sprinting to first base or a basketball player passing the ball, then cutting to the basket).

PUSH-UP & SPRINT

This exercise requires less thinking and more instinctive reaction. By beginning from a push-up position, you eliminate the leverage offered by a traditional start position, and you short-circuit the inclination to overanalyze takeoff and first steps. Instead, you scramble to your feet, then let instinct guide you through the first 10 yards of acceleration. After 1–2 reps, you'll find that you've adopted proper acceleration mechanics—from a good forward lean to the correct neuromuscular coordination for push-off.

132

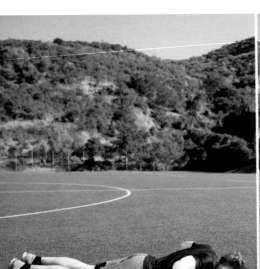
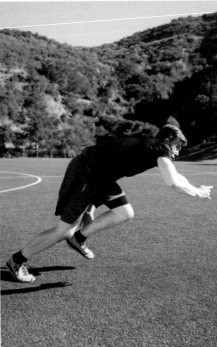
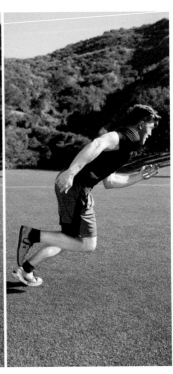

WORKOUT   **2–3 reps of 10–15 yards acceleration**

▸ Begin in a down push-up position.

▸ Scramble to your feet.

▸ Accelerate forward immediately (i.e., as soon as balance and body position allow).

STANDING STARTS

Almost all team-sports athletes will be called upon to accelerate from a standing start—and you won't just accelerate forward, but also laterally (I'm looking at you, baseball players). This drill prepares your nervous system to command powerful and efficient acceleration mechanics, regardless of which foot is forward or which direction you go.

133

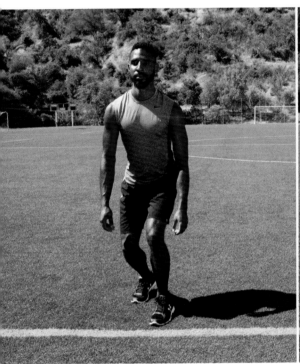
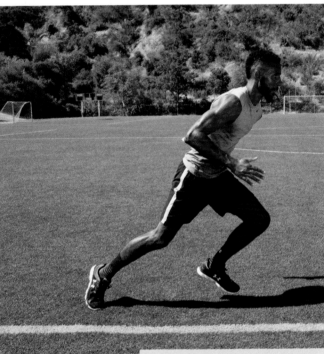

WORKOUT   1 set of the standing-start six pack (6 sprints)

▶ Begin in a standing start stance (see box).

▶ On command (external or internal), sprint 10 yards.

▶ Complete 6 sprints (your six pack) as follows, resting for 30 seconds between starts/sprints:

1/ Left foot forward, sprint forward 10 yards

2/ Right foot forward, sprint forward 10 yards

3/ Left foot forward, sprint to your left 10 yards (shown)

4/ Right foot forward, sprint to your right 10 yards

5/ Both feet even, sprint to the right 10 yards

6/ Both feet even, sprint to the left 10 yards

STANDING-START STANCE

▶ One leg forward, your other leg ½ to 1 foot length back

▶ Feet hip-width apart

▶ Knees bent, with a slight forward body lean

▶ Arms held loosely at your sides or with one arm forward, 90° bend at the elbow, and the other back (if your left leg is forward, your right arm should be forward)

STANDING 5-JUMP (OR 10-JUMP)

Acceleration is all about horizontal force. And the Standing 5-Jump is all about stringing together all-out, explosive, horizontal movement that will translate to powerful initial acceleration. This exercise puts the stretch-shortening cycles for your acceleration muscles into hyperdrive.

134

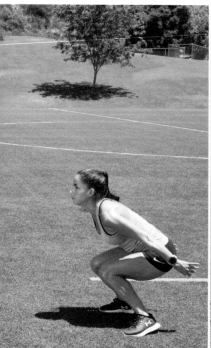
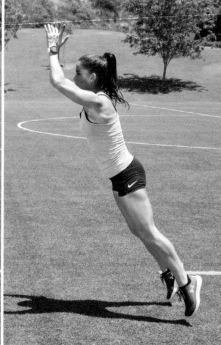
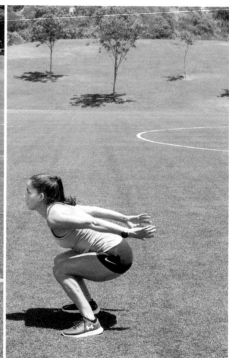

WORKOUT   **2 sets of 5–10 consecutive jumps**

▸ Stand with your feet hip-width apart, then squat, drawing your arms behind you.

▸ Jump forward as far as you can.

▸ Immediately drop into another squat, then spring forward with another jump. Repeat until you reach 5 jumps. As fitness improves, build up to 10 jumps.

COACH'S 2 CENTS

While your goal is to jump forward as far as you can, remember that you must land with enough stability to transition into the next squat and jump. In other words, jump as far as you can while maintaining balance and control.

WEIGHT SLED PUSH

If there's one exercise that benefits first-steps acceleration, it's the sled push. You'll work the big muscles (e.g., quadriceps and glutes) that drive acceleration, and you'll engage your back and core to maintain stability. Tackle this exercise early in the workout, when your legs are strong and your fatigue minimal.

135

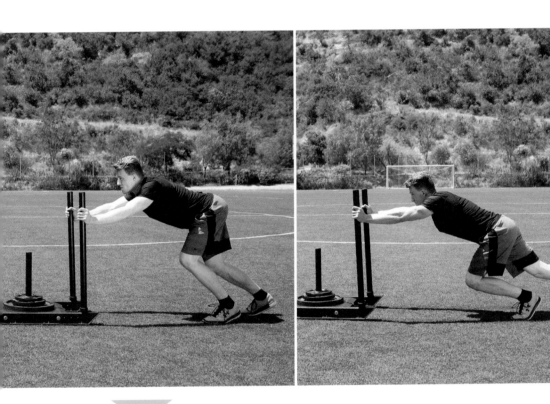

WORKOUT   **2 sets of 10–20 yards**

▶ Load the sled with the desired weight—from as little as 10% of your body weight to as much weight as you can handle.

▶ Line up behind the sled, hands on the handles, arms fully extended. Your feet should be 2–3 feet behind the sled, one foot slightly ahead of the other.

▶ Drive forward off your front foot. Angle your body up to 45° for leverage, with your knees bending 90° with each step forward, mimicking the angle you'll use for first-steps sprint acceleration. Keep eyes focused in front of the sled.

▶ Drive again . . . and again.

COACH'S 2 CENTS

Coach Mike Boyle writes, "In running speed, all the force production is from hip hyperextension. The ability to apply force to the ground and create forward movement can only occur when the foot is placed under the center of mass and pushed back . . . A weighted sled teaches strong athletes how to produce the type of force that moves them forward."

WEIGHT SLED MARCHING

Sled marching is a special strength exercise; it includes the same basic joint dynamics of sprinting but not the exact same neuromuscular activation sequence. With special strength training, preserving good acceleration form isn't a concern. That means you can load up on weight, with speedsters often using loads greater than 30 percent of body weight (BW). This is a terrific exercise for all phases of acceleration, from first steps to final steps.

136

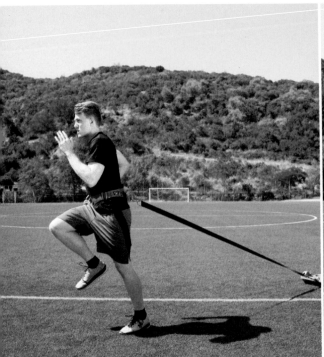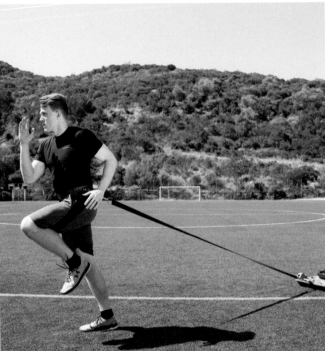

WORKOUT   2–3 sets of 15–20 yards (loads > 30% BW)
or 2–3 sets of 15–30 yards (loads < 30% BW)

▸ Load the sled with the desired weight. (Start light; you can go heavier later.)

▸ Stand so the tether between you and the weight sled is tight.

▸ March forward, driving one knee high while pushing off with the opposite leg. Extend your hip, knee, and ankle while pressing the ball of your foot into the ground, keeping your elbows bent at about 90°.

▸ Synchronize arm swings with knee lifts: left knee up with right arm forward, right knee up with left arm forward.

COACH'S 2 CENTS

This isn't about speed; it's about getting into a nice rhythm and driving forward with the down leg—don't be afraid to really come up on the ball of your foot. Also, a waist harness (versus a shoulder harness) allows you to apply force in a more natural way.

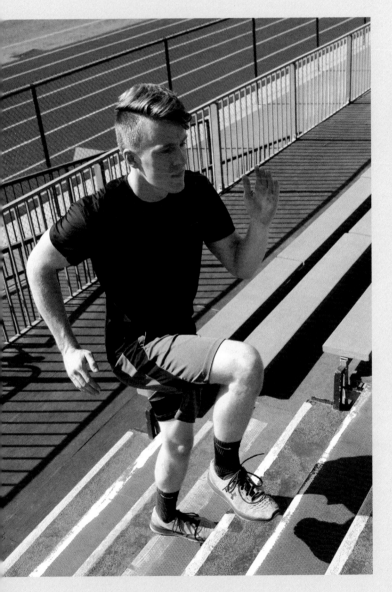

No-prop alternative:
STADIUM STEPS (MARCHING)

If you don't have a weight sled, you can get a similar workout on your local school's stadium steps:

▸ Start at the base of the steps, then march up the steps, lifting one knee high and then using the same-side foot to land on the next step—climb 1–2 steps at a time, depending on the depth and height of the steps.

▸ Synchronize arm swing to knee lift (right to left, and left to right) and keep your elbows at 90°.

▸ Start with 10 marching steps total, then build up as fitness dictates.

WEIGHT SLED RUN

This exercise develops horizontal force for the transition phase of acceleration. It's a specific strength exercise, mimicking the neuromuscular activation sequence of unresisted acceleration sprinting. That means you'll need to accelerate at a minimum of 90 percent of your unresisted pace, while maintaining the same form you'd employ for unresisted acceleration. The traditional load for this exercise is 10-15 percent of body weight, but studies have shown that greater acceleration benefits can be had at heavier loads—that said, don't overload the sled, as you won't benefit from work performed with substandard form.

138

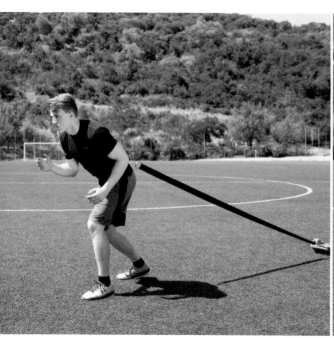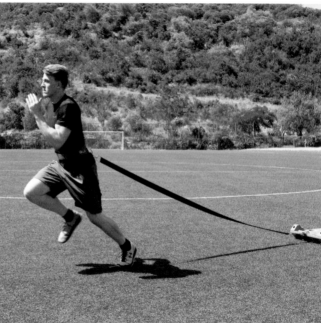

WORKOUT   **2-3 reps of 15-20 yards**

▶ Load the sled with your desired weight—try 10-15% of body weight, and adjust as your form and pace dictate.

▶ Begin with the tether stretched tight between you and the weight sled.

▶ Accelerate to 90-95% of your unresisted speed, using the first 2-3 steps to build into your pace.

COACH'S 2 CENTS

A sled with a larger surface area on the bottom is less likely to flip while being dragged. Also, a waist harness (versus a shoulder harness) allows you to apply force in a more natural way.

AGILITY
TRAINING

AGILITY LADDER 1-LEGGED HOPS

This drill combines the most basic plyometric movement—the hop—with the mechanical constraints presented by an agility ladder. You'll exploit elastic recoil to power short, controlled, direction- and distance-specific hops.

140

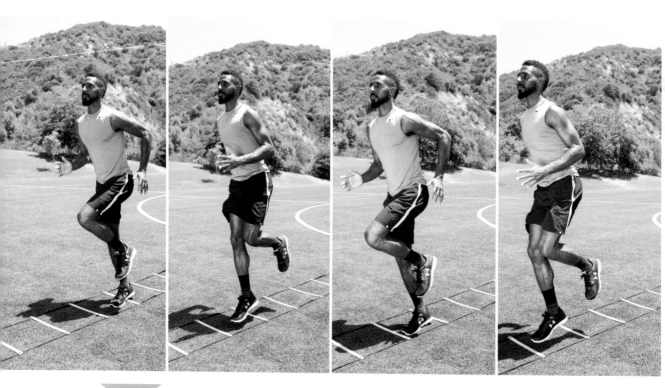

WORKOUT **1 rep with each leg (2 reps total) of the entire ladder**

▶ Step into the first ladder unit (the space between the first and second rungs) with one foot.

▶ Then immediately hop using the same foot into the next ladder unit.

▶ Continue hopping on one foot from one ladder unit to the next. As you hop, move your arms to counterbalance your leg movement.

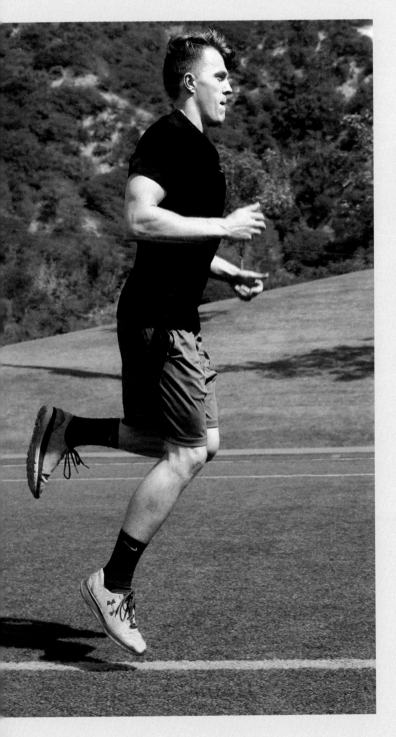

No-prop alternative:

1-LEGGED HOPS

If you don't have an agility ladder, you can still perform 1-Legged Hops:

▶ Balance on one foot.

▶ Hop forward, limiting your hops to 12–14 inches, for 10 hops total. If you have access to a marked line, perform the exercise using that line as a guide.

AGILITY LADDER 2-LEGGED HOPS

Two-legged hopping is a great dual-purpose drill. First, you'll develop nervous-system efficiency for the types of short, quick movements required in sports like basketball, tennis, and football. Second, it's a great stimulus for improving controlled, horizontal-force explosiveness.

142

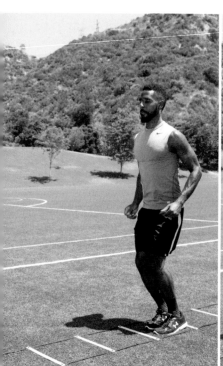
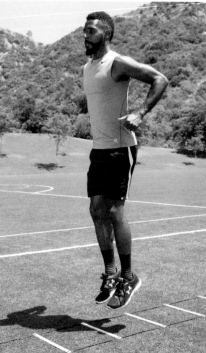
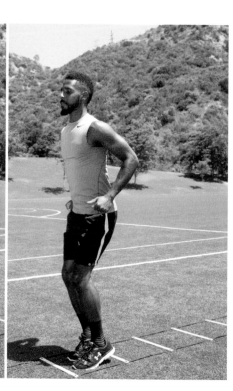

▼ **WORKOUT** **1–2 reps of the entire ladder**

▸ Stand directly behind the ladder, feet hip-width apart.

▸ Jump over the first ladder unit (the space between the first and second rungs) landing on both feet in the second ladder unit. Quickly hop with both feet, landing in the fourth ladder unit.

▸ Continue hopping with both feet, skipping one ladder unit with each hop.

COACH'S 2 CENTS

Don't dawdle after landing; let your knees bend slightly, then quickly transition to the next hop. Also, look at the ladder! This isn't about memorizing the distance between rungs (i.e., this isn't a proprioception drill); it's about controlled horizontal force.

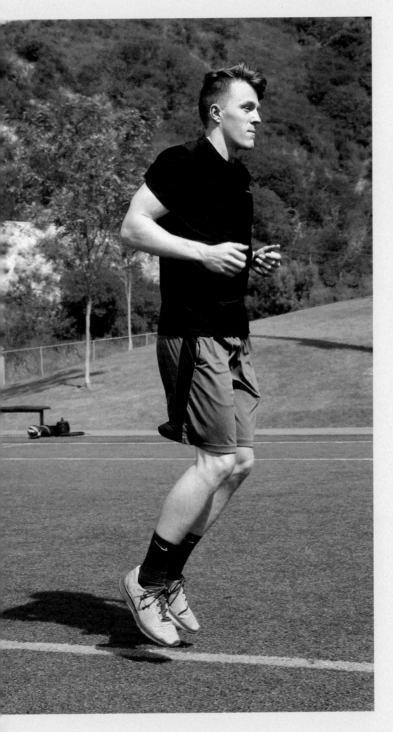

No-prop alternative:
2-LEGGED HOPS

If you don't have an agility ladder, you can still perform 2-Legged Hops:

▶ Stand with your feet parallel, hip-width apart.

▶ Hop forward with both feet, limiting your hops to 12–24 inches, for 10 hops total. If you have access to a marked line, perform the exercise using that line as a guide.

AGILITY LADDER 3 QUICK STEPS

You'll emphasize quick foot plant and rapid leg movement in this nervous-system drill. This is the agility ladder version of 3-Step, 1-Step.

144

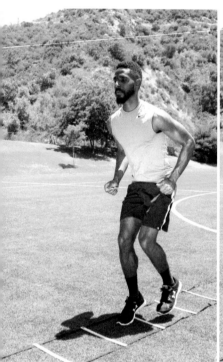 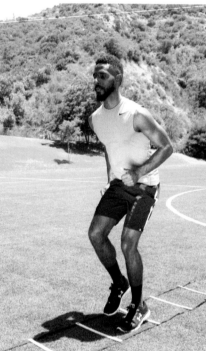 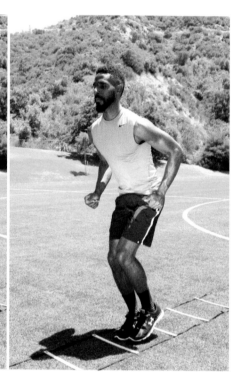

WORKOUT **1–2 reps of the entire ladder**

▶ Stand behind the ladder, feet no more than hip-width apart.

▶ Step into the first ladder unit (the space between the first and second rungs) with your right foot. Quickly follow with your left foot, then do a quick step-in-place in the same ladder unit with your right foot.

▶ Step forward into the second ladder unit with your left foot. Quickly follow with your right foot, then do another quick step-in-place in the same ladder unit with your left foot.

▶ Repeat the process of three quick steps in each ladder unit, alternating the foot you step with first.

COACH'S 2 CENTS

Don't be discouraged if you have trouble keeping count—"1-2-3"—and then alternating feet as you step into each successive ladder unit. This is a drill that your body will learn through practice—in other words, don't think your way through this drill, just do it.

AGILITY LADDER ICKEY SHUFFLE

"Ickey" Woods was a fullback with the NFL's Cincinnati Bengals who made headlines for his post-touchdown celebration dance, the Ickey Shuffle. Former teammate Boomer Esiason says of the dance, "I don't know what he was drinking the day he came up with it, but it was a sensation throughout the 1988 season." Considered so bad that it was good, the dance inspired this drill (or maybe vice versa), which targets quick foot plant, lateral movement, and lower leg coordination.

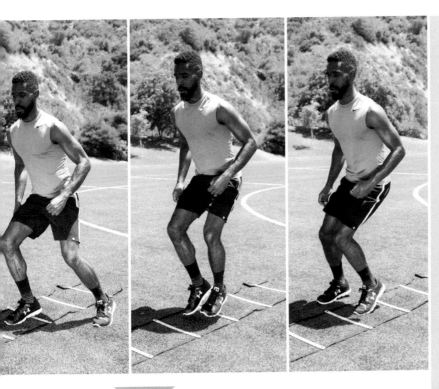

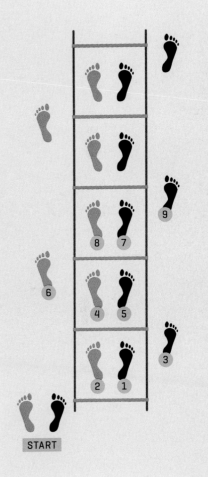

WORKOUT **1–2 reps of the entire ladder**

▸ Stand to the left of the ladder's first rung, your feet close together.

▸ Step into the first ladder unit (the space between the first and second rungs) with your right foot. Quickly place your left foot in the ladder unit next to your right foot. Step outside the ladder—to the right—with your right foot.

▸ Step into the second ladder unit with your left foot. Quickly place your right foot in the ladder unit next to your left foot. Step outside the ladder—to the left—with your left foot.

▸ Continue Ickey-shuffling the length of the ladder.

AGILITY LADDER STEP IN 'N' OUT

This straightforward stepping drill teaches your nervous system to command quick movement in a horizontal (forward and backward) direction, which is essential for defensive play in many sports. This is the agility ladder version of the Step Back 'n' Forth Drill.

146

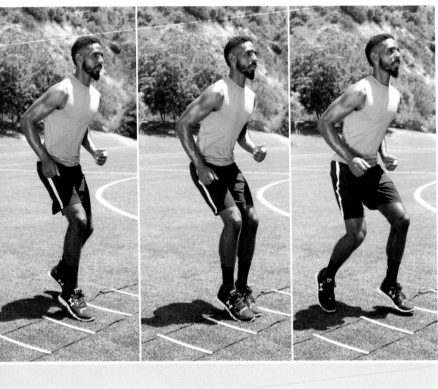

1 rep of the ladder in each direction (2 reps total)

▸ Stand beside the ladder, facing it, with your feet hip-width apart.

▸ Step into the first ladder unit (the space between the first and second rungs) with your right foot. Quickly place your left foot into the same unit, next to your right foot.

▸ Step back with your right foot, setting it down in front of the second ladder unit. Step back with your left foot, setting it down next to the right foot.

▸ Repeat the previous steps, beginning with a right-foot step into the second ladder unit.

▸ For your second rep, begin at the opposite end of the ladder (staying on the same side as your first rep), then step first with your left foot and move to your left down the ladder.

STEP BACK 'N' FORTH DRILL

This simple stepping drill teaches your nervous system to command quick movement in a horizontal (forward and backward) direction, which is essential for defensive play in many sports. If you have an agility ladder, you can perform the Step In 'n' Out version of this drill.

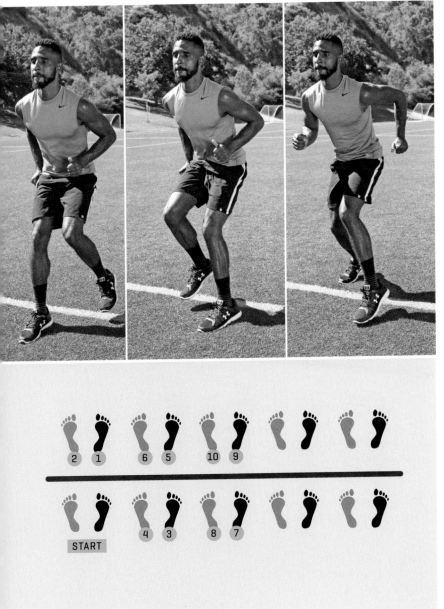

▼ **WORKOUT** 1 rep each direction (2 reps total) of 10–15 yards

▶ Stand with feet hip-width apart, toes on one side of a marked line on a field—(if there is no line, create or imagine one).

▶ Step over the line with your right foot. Quickly place your left foot over the line next to your right foot. Step back diagonally (to the right) with your right foot, setting it down in front of the line. Step back with your left foot, setting it down next to your right foot.

▶ Repeat the previous steps as you move down the line.

▶ For your second rep, begin at the opposite end of the line (facing the same direction as on your first rep), then step first with your left foot and move left down the line.

3-STEP, 1-STEP

This nervous-system drill emphasizes quick foot plant and rapid leg movement. You can perform it anywhere, although some athletes prefer a marked line to track forward progress. If you have an agility ladder, you can perform the 3 Quick Steps version of this drill (see page 144).

148

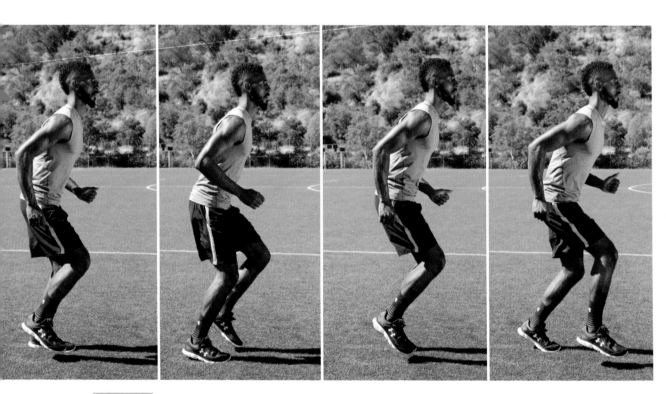

WORKOUT   **1–2 sets of 10–15 yards**

▸ Stand with your feet hip-width apart, arms at your sides, elbows bent.

▸ Step forward with your right foot. Quickly move your left foot next to your right foot. Lift your right foot up and down, stepping in place.

▸ Step forward with your left foot. Quickly move your right foot next to your left foot. Lift your left foot up and down, stepping in place.

▸ Repeat the pattern: Step forward, follow with the opposite foot, step-in-place with the first foot, then step forward again with the opposite foot.

COACH'S 2 CENTS

Don't worry about how quickly you do this drill on your first attempt. The key is to nail the cadence, then improve how quickly you perform that cadence from rep to rep.

SIDE STEPS (QUICK)

Developing lateral quickness requires rewiring your nervous system to better control the muscles that drive lateral motion—namely, hip abductors and hip adductors. This drill helps you do that rewiring, as well as work on balance and proprioception.

149

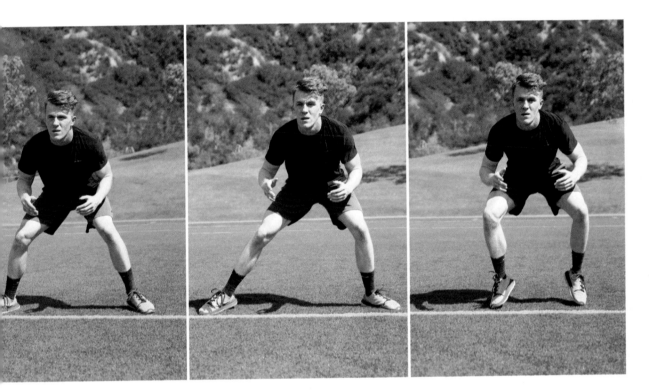

WORKOUT **1–2 reps each direction (2–4 reps total) for 15–20 yards**

▶ Begin with your feet hip-width apart, knees bent, arms held out from your sides, elbows slightly bent.

▶ Step sideways with your left foot while driving off your right foot. Quickly lift your right foot to recreate the original distance between your feet. As your right foot lands, immediately step left again, driving with your right foot.

▶ After completing a rep in one direction, lead with your right foot for a second rep in the opposite direction.

COACH'S 2 CENTS

Move quickly through this drill. Fast action is essential. But also focus on stability and balance. Some athletes (e.g., football linebackers) should ensure there's no "hop" as they plant their drive foot before stepping to the side; other athletes, for whom quickness is valued more highly than stability, can incorporate a slight hop into the movement.

BACKWARD RUNNING

Backward running plays an essential role in many sports. Whether you're fading to catch a pop fly in baseball, backing up to defend a receiver in football, or backpedaling after draining a shot in basketball, this is a skill you need to master.

150

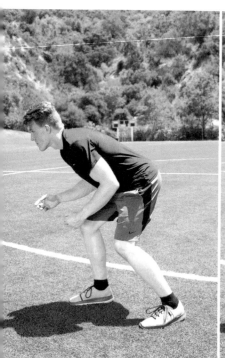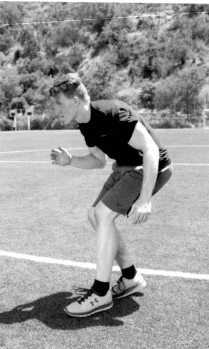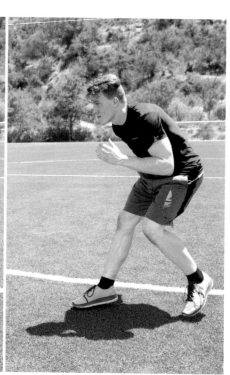

WORKOUT 2 sets of 20–30 yards

- Start with knees bent, one foot slightly behind the other (weight distributed slightly more to the forward foot), elbows bent and hands held low.

- Push backward—don't bound—while maintaining your starting posture.

- Go as fast as you can while maintaining the ability to alter direction at any point.

- If training with a partner, take turns calling out changes in direction (forward, lateral, or a 180° turn). This allows you to mimic reactions you'll make as a defender on the field or court.

COACH'S 2 CENTS

Your prime goal is to maintain balance and stability. Even if you train alone, incorporate changes of direction into your backpedaling. While you won't practice the quick reaction demanded of defenders, you'll teach your body how to execute changes of direction from a backward gait.

MINI-SUICIDES

This fun exercise is great for finishing off a workout, and it's also good for a little competition if you're training with a friend. This is a shortened version of the more intense "suicides" that athletes have experienced and dreaded for ages. With mini-suicides, it's less about speed endurance (the traditional suicides' target) and more about start-and-stop agility.

151

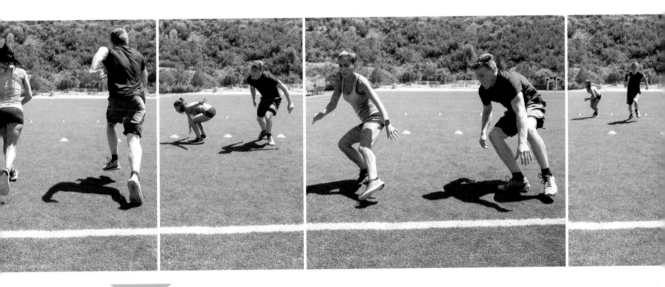

WORKOUT   1–3 reps

▶ Begin from a standing start at the start line.

▶ Sprint forward 5 yards and touch the ground with your right hand. Sprint back to the start line and touch down with your left hand. Sprint forward 10 yards and touch down with your right hand. Sprint back through the start line to finish.

COACH'S 2 CENTS

If you're training with a partner, feel free to introduce a little competition into this exercise. Race each other: best two out of three.

BALANCE ON 1 LEG

Simple can be powerful. Balancing on one leg is one of the most effective ways to improve overall balance, as your nervous system is forced to make constant adjustments in muscle tension and contraction from head to toe. A 2007 study found that football players who balanced on each leg for five minutes, five days a week, for four weeks during preseason, sustained 77 percent fewer ankle sprains during the season.

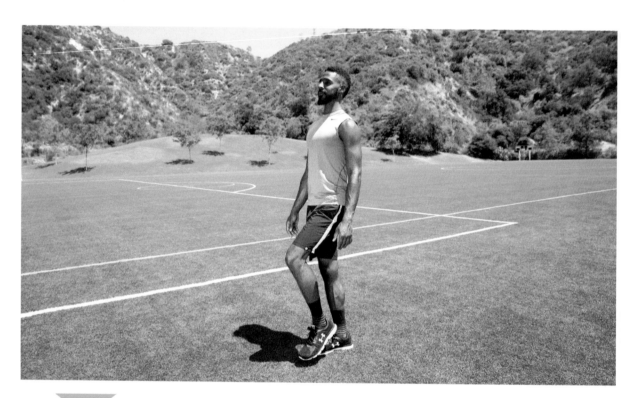

WORKOUT 1 set of 30 seconds on each foot

▶ Stand with your knees slightly bent, arms loose at your sides.

▶ Lift one foot in front of you, a few inches off the ground. Hold it there for 30 seconds—less if you can't maintain balance.

▶ Switch feet.

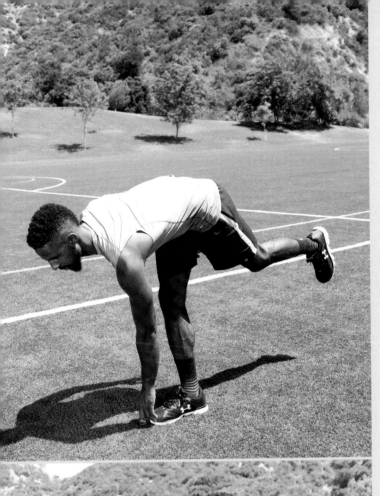

Additional instruction for
ADDING A TOE TOUCH

▶ Once the exercise is mastered, add a controlled toe touch.

▶ Swing your lifted foot behind you.

▶ Bend down to touch your toes (or as close as you can get) with your opposite-side hand.

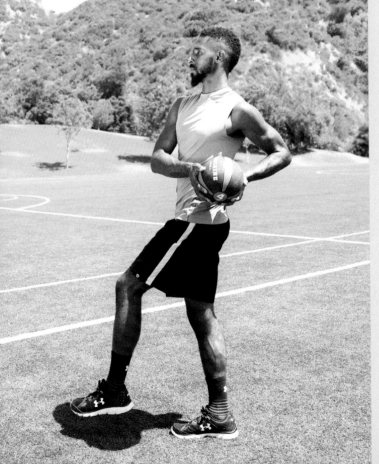

Additional instruction for
ADDING A MEDBALL

▶ Begin in the balance position with a medball held in front of your chest.

▶ Lift the medball over your head, move it side-to-side, or bend down to touch it to the ground.

20-YARD SQUARE AND 40-YARD SQUARE

This drill not only requires you to change direction, it also requires that you change your method of locomotion. You'll run forward, backward, and sideways, practicing quick transitions between each. Being able to execute these transitions is essential in sports like football, tennis, and basketball.

154

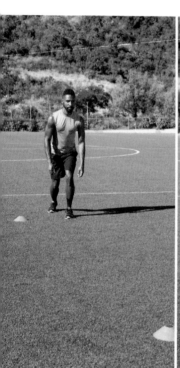
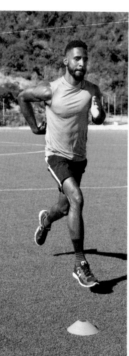
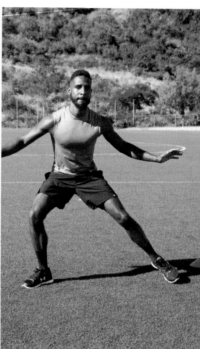
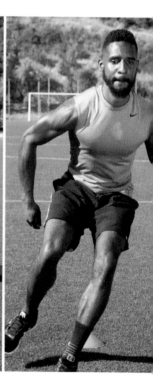

WORKOUT 1–2 reps of the course

▸ Begin from a standing start [page 133] just outside the lower-left cone.

▸ Accelerate forward to the upper-left cone.

▸ Transition to a side shuffle, traveling right toward the upper-right cone.

▸ At the upper-right cone, transition to backward running, aiming for the outside of the lower-right cone.

▸ At the lower-right cone, transition into a side shuffle, traveling left to the lower-left cone.

▸ For the second rep, begin from the lower-right cone and reverse directions.

COACH'S 2 CENTS

When the 20-yard square gets easy, try a 40-yard square (10 yards on each side), but make sure you've mastered your transitions before moving up to the longer distance.

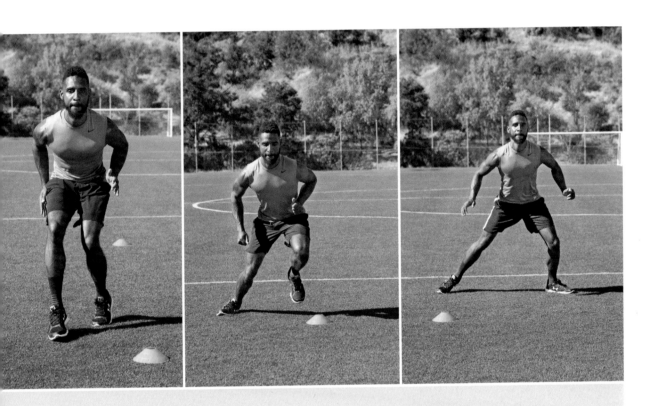

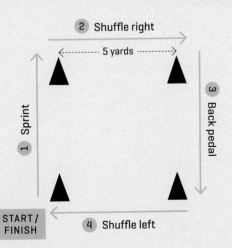

COURSE SET-UP
Use 4 cones (or prop swaps)
for the four corners of
a square. Each side of the
square should measure
5 yards.

2 Shuffle right

<----- 5 yards ----->

1 Sprint

3 Back pedal

START /
FINISH

4 Shuffle left

FIGURE 8 DRILL

This is a great drill for hardwiring your neuromuscular system for changes of direction, quick pivoting, and acceleration/deceleration skills. It's also fun! That makes it a perfect drill to cap off a training session.

156

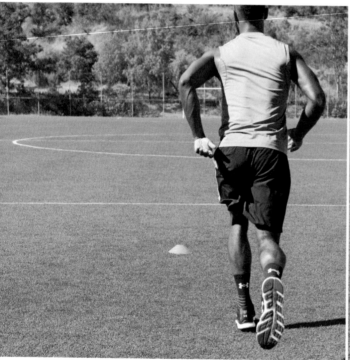
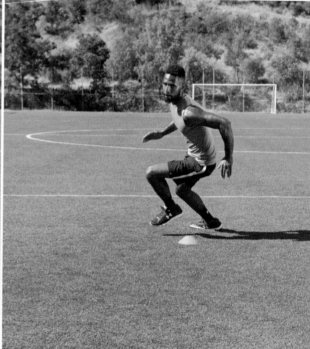

WORKOUT **2 reps**

▸ Begin with your left foot to the right of the start cone.

▸ Sprint straight ahead to the right side of the second cone, bending at the waist as you cut left around it.

▸ Sprint diagonally back toward the right side (the side you started on) of the start cone, bending at the waist as you cut right around it.

▸ Sprint straight ahead toward the left side of the second cone. That cone is your finish line.

COACH'S 2 CENTS

If you don't have cones, use a prop swap—even an old pair of shoes will do.

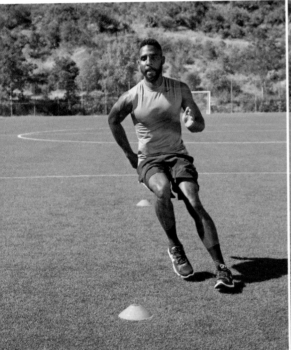

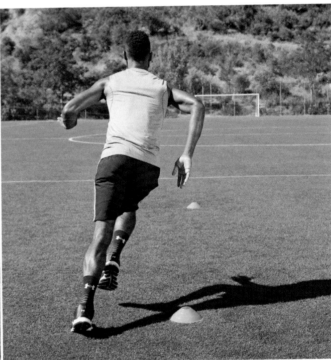

COURSE SETUP
Place two cones (or similar props)
5 yards apart.

FINISH

5 yards

START

Additional instruction for
FIGURE 8 DRILL
WITH A PARTNER:

▸ Set the cones 10 yards apart
instead of 5.

▸ Start with your partner 3 yards
behind you.

▸ Do the drill as instructed. You
decide when to start, and your partner
reacts by chasing you. If your partner
catches you, he or she wins. Change
start positions and go again.

W-PATTERN CONE DRILL

This one is all about controlled agility and acceleration. It isn't a drill where you go 100 percent from the start. Instead, you'll use sub-maximum acceleration and focus on fluid turns and good form.

158

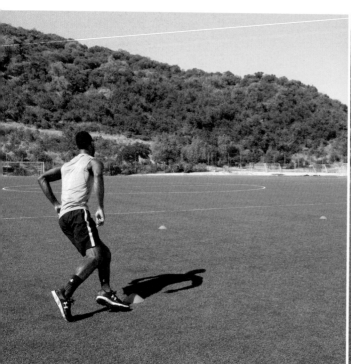
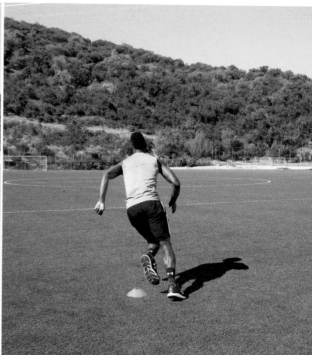

COURSE SETUP

Use 5 cones (or prop swaps) to form an upside-down "W" pattern. Place 3 cones on one line, 5 yards apart—the first cone on that line is cone 1, with cones 3 and 5 to its right. On a line 5 yards ahead of the first line, set up 2 more cones, also 5 yards apart, located directly between the cones on the first line—the first cone on that line is cone 2, with cone 4 to its right.

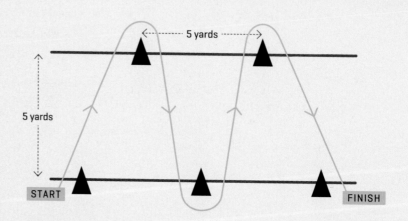

5 yards

5 yards

START

FINISH

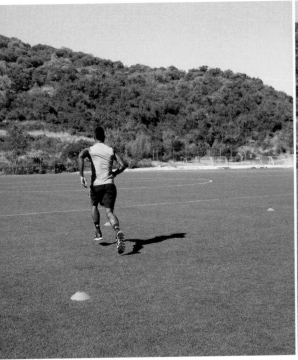 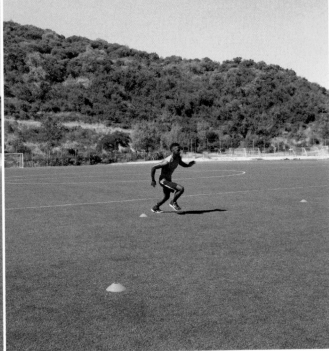

WORKOUT   **1 rep each direction (2 reps total) of the course**

▶ Start with your right foot on the outside of cone 1.

▶ Accelerate at 80 to 90% effort toward cone 2. Bend at the waist and cut right around cone 2 and accelerate toward cone 3. Bend at the waist and cut left around cone 3 and accelerate toward cone 4. Bend at the waist and cut right around cone 4, then accelerate to finish at cone 5.

▶ After a 1–2-minute recovery, repeat in the opposite direction.

COACH'S 2 CENTS

Run at 80–90% effort for this drill. The slower pace allows you to focus on change of direction. Maximum speed isn't your goal.

WEIGHT SLED CROSSOVER

With this exercise, you'll put the burn to your hip abductors and hip adductors. Since both muscle groups are major players when it comes to stabilizing horizontal movement, you'll also shore up your sprint form stability.

160

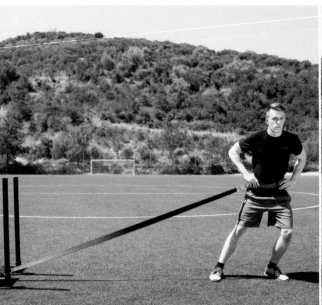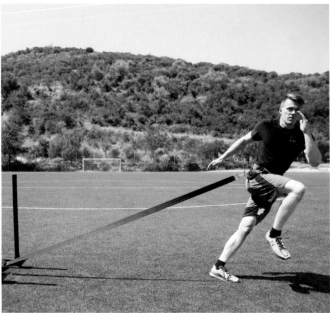

WORKOUT   **2–3 reps of 10–15 yards**

▸ Load the sled with weight—from as little as 10% of your body weight to as much weight as you can handle.

▸ Stand to the left of the sled, and lean left, bending your left leg at the knee while keeping your right leg straight. The tether should be taut.

▸ Lift your right leg, bending at the knee, and bring it across the front of your left leg. Simultaneously straighten your left leg to exert lateral force against the ground.

▸ After landing your right leg, straighten it to keep moving sideways. Bend your left leg and cross over behind your right leg, recreating your original stance.

▸ Repeat this crossover pattern for the remainder of the rep. After your first rep, rest 1–2 minutes, then repeat in the opposite direction, switching which leg crosses in front and which leg crosses behind.

COACH'S 2 CENTS

It's important to work both legs equally during each rep, as the leg crossing in front works abductors, while the leg crossing behind works adductors. If possible, use a waist harness rather than a shoulder harness. A waist harness keeps the resistance closer to your center of mass and makes it easier to maintain proper form.

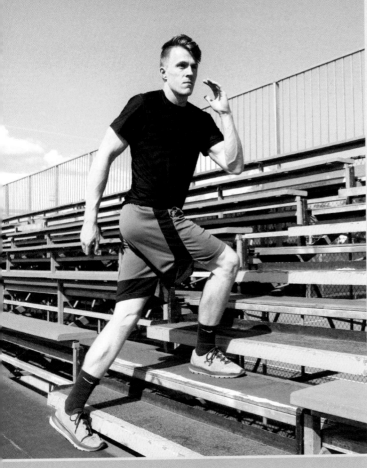

No-prop alternative:

STADIUM CROSSOVER STEPS

If you don't have a weight sled, you can get a similar workout on your local school's stadium steps:

▶ Begin at the base of the steps, then utilize the same crossover instructions as listed for the Weight Sled Crossover to begin climbing the steps, moving sideways.

▶ Climb 1 or 2 steps at a time, depending on the depth/height of the steps and your fitness.

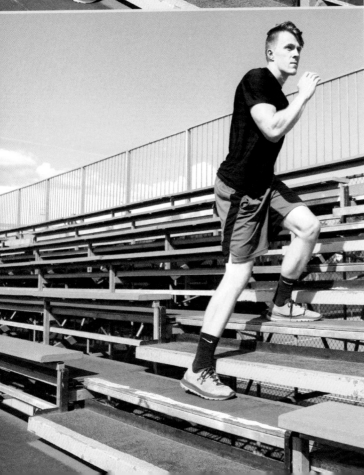

MAXIMUM VELOCITY TRAINING

SKIPPING

This is the same schoolyard skipping you remember from childhood. Skipping stimulates elastic recoil and helps teach your body to "pop" off your toes with each stride. It also serves as a great warm up for the drills that follow.

164

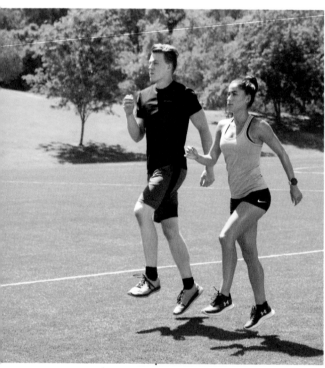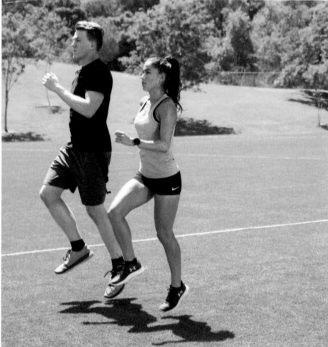

WORKOUT   **1 rep of 20-60 yards**

▸ Step forward with your right foot and spring vertically and horizontally, landing on the same (right) foot.

▸ Next, step forward with your left foot, and spring vertically and horizontally, landing on the same (left) foot.

▸ Step forward with your right foot, and continue the pattern.

▸ After completing the drill, jog back to your start line, then immediately perform a stride at 90% effort (same distance as drill), followed by a walk back to the start line.

HIGH SKIPPING

This variation of skipping allows you to direct force in a vertical direction, while exaggerating concentric calf contribution and knee lift.

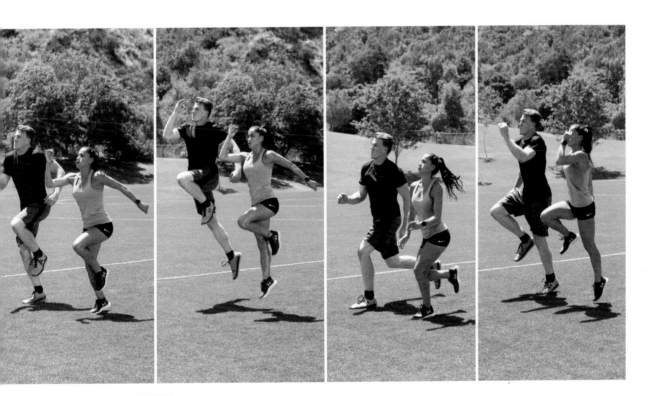

WORKOUT   **1 rep of 20–60 yards**

▶ Step forward with your right foot and spring vertically off the ball of that foot, swinging your right arm in an exaggerated arc (your hand should end up near your forehead). Simultaneously lift your left knee high.

▶ Land on the same (right) foot, and then step forward with your left foot. Spring vertically off that foot, while lifting your right knee and left arm.

▶ Land on your left foot, step forward with your right foot, and continue the pattern.

▶ After completing the drill, jog back to your start line, then immediately perform a stride at 90% effort (same distance as drill), followed by a walk back to the start line.

COACH'S 2 CENTS

The goal is to get good height on each skip, not to move forward rapidly.

FLAT-FOOTED MARCHING

"Knee lift position" largely controls how hard your foot hits the ground (by determining the distance you accelerate your foot downward)—and as you recall from Chapter 4, the key to maximum velocity is to hit the ground hard. This drill teaches your hip extensors "reduced inhibition" (a science-y way of saying less opposition from your glutes and hamstrings) while simultaneously training those same muscles to allow greater range of motion (i.e., a higher knee lift). That's double-good news for knee lift.

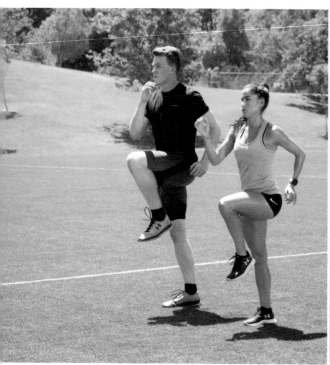 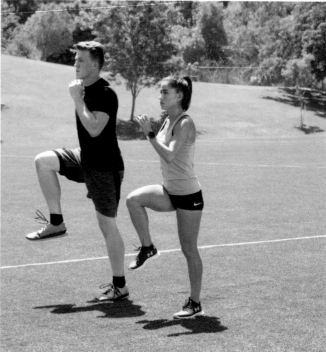

WORKOUT **1 rep of 20–60 yards**

▶ March forward, lifting your right knee to waist-height or higher, maintaining a 90° angle at your ankle (in other words, don't point your foot).

▶ Bring your right foot down, actively accelerating it toward the ground without stomping the ground. Land flatfooted, and then repeat with your left leg.

▶ Continue alternating legs, moving your arms in a running motion throughout the drill.

▶ After completing the drill, jog back to your start line, then immediately perform a stride at 90% effort (same distance as drill), followed by a walk back to the start line.

HIGH KNEES

This drill targets your neuromuscular system and works two key aspects of maximum velocity: elastic recoil and knee lift. First, you drive the ball of your foot into the ground, generating a high vertical force that results in equally large elastic energy storage in your Achilles and arch. Next, you release this energy to fuel your leg's bounce back to high knee lift position, at which point a stretch reflex in your glutes and hamstrings slingshots your thigh in the reverse direction.

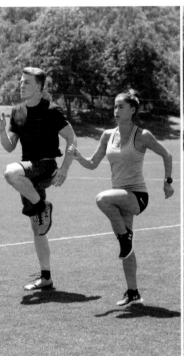
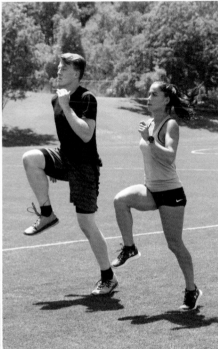
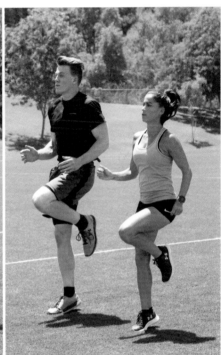

WORKOUT **1 rep of 20–60 yards**

▸ After jogging a few steps, drive your right knee upward.

▸ Forcefully bring your right leg down (don't just let it fall), landing on the ball of your foot. Simultaneously lift your left knee.

▸ Press your landing foot down until your heel almost taps the ground, then allow elastic recoil from your Achilles and arch to fuel a "bounce" as you drive your knee to waist height or better. As one knee rises, the opposite foot comes down.

▸ After completing the drill, jog back to your start line, then immediately perform a stride at 90% effort (same distance as drill), followed by a walk back to the start line.

COACH'S 2 CENTS

Keep your legs moving quickly during this drill, with all the action on your "front side" (i.e., work your legs in front of your body). Some athletes find leaning backward helps maintain stability and increase knee lift. Stay on the balls of your feet throughout the drill and work your arms.

QUICK FEET

This drill does double duty for your training. You'll practice reduced contact time for maximum velocity, while simultaneously training foot speed for agility. You'll also give your tibialis anterior and peroneal group (outside calf) muscles a solid workout— if you do this drill correctly, those muscles will be burning.

168

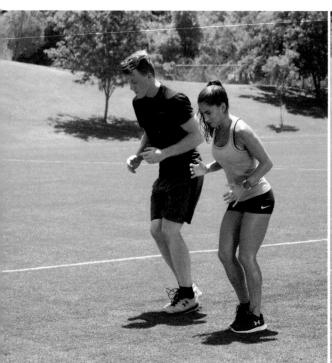
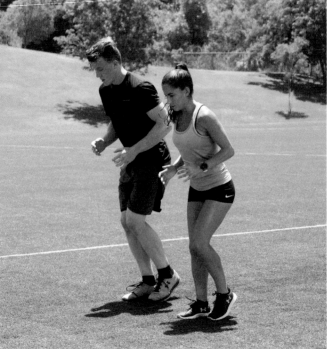

WORKOUT   1 rep of 20–30 yards

▶ Begin with your feet hip-width apart, elbows bent at 90° and held loosely at your sides.

▶ Lift your right foot and quickly step forward a few inches. The bottom of your shoe should not rise more than 1–3 inches off the ground.

▶ Repeat with your left foot, and then with your right foot, etc., shuffling as quickly as you can for 20–30 yards.

▶ After completing the drill, jog back to your start line, then immediately perform a stride at 90% effort (same distance as drill), followed by a walk back to the start line.

COACH'S 2 CENTS

Don't try to sync your arm movement with your quick leg movement—equally quick arm movement would disrupt your balance and rhythm. Some runners find that a slow-motion approximation of running arm swing works well.

QUICK HOPS

This plyometric drill is perfect for practicing the quick bursts of combined vertical and horizontal force you'll need to produce at maximum velocity. Some athletes call these bunny hops. But don't let the cute name fool you. These deliver a major burn to your quads. If you start losing form—and it goes quick with this drill—it's time to jog back to the start line.

169

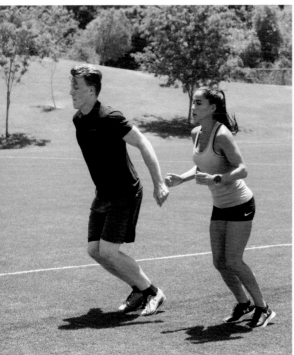 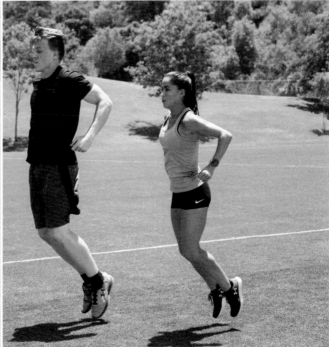

WORKOUT   **1 rep of 20–30 yards**

▶ Begin with your feet hip-width apart, elbows at 90°, arms at your sides (see "Coach's 2 Cents" for more on arm carriage).

▶ Spring forward with both feet, focusing on horizontal—not vertical—motion. Keep your jumps low to the ground (a few inches' clearance is fine).

▶ As soon as you land, jump again, keeping a quick rhythm as you hop for the remainder of the drill.

▶ After completing the drill, jog back to your start line and immediately perform a stride at 90% effort (same distance as drill), followed by a walk back to the start line.

COACH'S 2 CENTS

As with Quick Feet, you'll have a hard time syncing your arms to your movement. Some runners draw both arms back as they jump, then push them forward when they land. Experiment to find what works best for your balance and stability.

BUTT KICKS

At maximum velocity, your heel rises toward your glutes due to a stretch reflex, forward momentum, and a hinge-like action at your knee, the latter of which allows force created by the former to swing your lower leg backward. So why perform a butt kicks drill that has a completely different genesis for movement, relying on the hamstrings' concentric contraction? One, because you'll strengthen muscles involved in butt-kicking, and two, because it increases your quadriceps' range of motion and sprint-readiness.

170

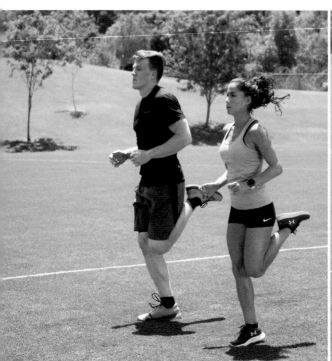
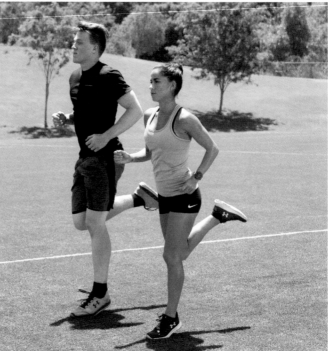

WORKOUT   **1 rep of 20–60 yards**

▸ Run tall, stay on the balls of your feet, and keep your thighs perpendicular to the ground as you quickly lift one heel toward your glutes—either touch or come as close as you can. Do the same with your opposite leg.

▸ Work your arms in a running motion throughout the drill.

▸ After completing the drill, jog back to the start line, then immediately perform a stride at 90% effort (same distance as drill), followed by a walk back to the start line.

COACH'S 2 CENTS

Don't kick back too hard with your leg—just use a quick, rhythmic movement. Also, the goal is quick butt kicking, not rapid forward locomotion.

STRAIGHT-LEG BOUNDING

This is a great exercise for activating your glutes (the muscle group that sprinters refer to as the engine) and your hamstrings (the muscle group most sprint researchers credit with driving maximum velocity). You'll also activate your quadriceps, making this an exercise that pays equal dividends for hip extension and hip flexion.

171

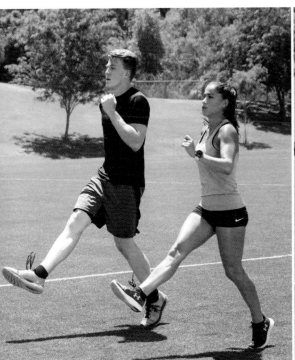
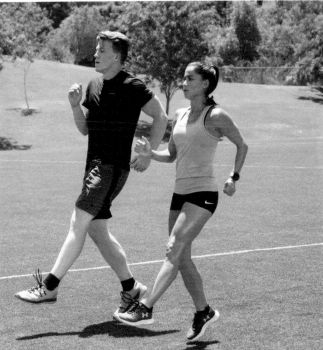

WORKOUT **1–2 reps of 20–40 yards**

▶ Begin with a few yards of jogging.

▶ Extend both legs fully at the knee (i.e., straighten your legs). Lift your right leg, utilizing your hip flexors. Simultaneously, drive down your left leg, using your glutes and hamstrings for a powerful hip extension.

▶ Be sure to land on the ball of your foot—stay off your heels throughout the exercise.

▶ Next, lift your left leg and drive down your right.

COACH'S 2 CENTS

This exercise can be worked into your maximum velocity drills or performed à la carte.

TRIPLE HOP ON 1 LEG

Triple hops are great for developing both vertical and horizontal force, key ingredients in maximum velocity.

172

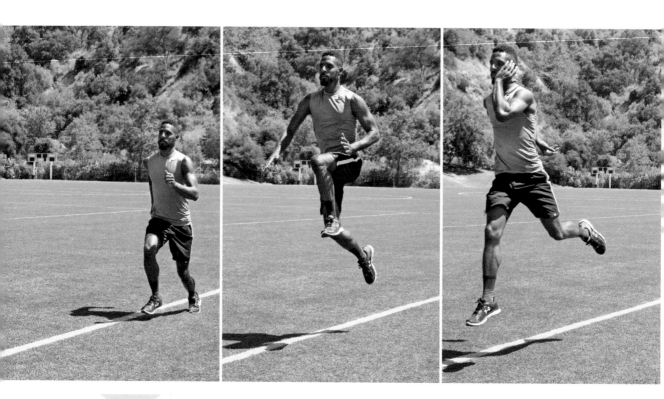

WORKOUT **2–3 reps for each foot**

▶ From a standing start, accelerate for 5 yards.

▶ Hop off your right foot as far as you can. Follow with two more hops off your right foot.

▶ Repeat the exercise hopping off your left foot.

COACH'S 2 CENTS

Don't worry about distance the first time you attempt this exercise. Instead, focus on execution. As you get more experienced, increase the distance of each hop. For balance, try pumping your arms back and forth while in the air.

DEPTH JUMP

If you had to pick one secret weapon for maximum velocity, this could be it. Dropping off a plyo box assures strong eccentric contractions upon landing, a powerful stretch-shortening cycle, oodles of stored elastic energy, and—if the transition time to concentric contraction is minimized—a maximal vertical explosion for the rebound jump. Multiple studies have shown a high correlation between depth-jump performance and leg stiffness, muscle stretch-shortening capacity, and flying 10-meter time.

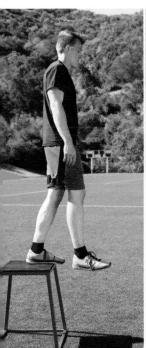 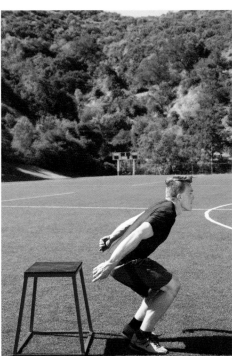 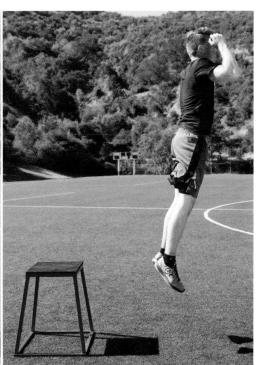

WORKOUT   3–5 reps

▸ Stand with your feet at the front edge of a plyo box (12–30 inches high).

▸ Step (don't jump) straight out from the box and let yourself drop.

▸ Land on both feet, letting your knees bend to absorb the force. Swing your arms behind your body as you land.

▸ Spring straight up (vertically)—not forward (horizontally).

COACH'S 2 CENTS

Transition quickly from landing to jump—the quicker this transition, the greater the release of energy when you jump. Also, since this is a powerful nervous system exercise, start with the minimum number of reps and don't add more than 1 rep per session.

JUMP SQUATS

The Jump Squat utilizes your stretch-shortening cycle. You'll create eccentric contractions of the quadriceps, hip extensors, and calves as you drop into a squat, and then trigger strong concentric contractions when you reverse direction with the jump. You'll improve your explosive vertical force, essential for both maximum velocity and the transition phase of acceleration.

174

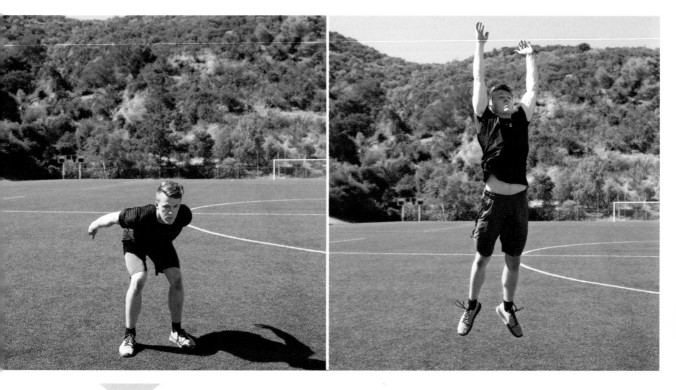

WORKOUT 1–2 sets of 5–10 reps

▶ With feet shoulder-width apart and toes pointed slightly outward, drop into a squat until your thighs are parallel to the ground (you can go lower, as your fitness improves and as your range of motion allows).

▶ Explode upward, bringing your arms forward and extending them over your head.

▶ As you land, drop back into the squat position.

▶ Immediately rebound with another jump.

COACH'S 2 CENTS

Extend your arms behind you as you squat, then swing them forward as you jump, adding to your vertical propulsion. Always jump straight up, as your injury risk is significantly higher when performing weighted jumps in a horizontal direction. Also, if using weight, a vest creates a more even distribution of weight than dumbbells.

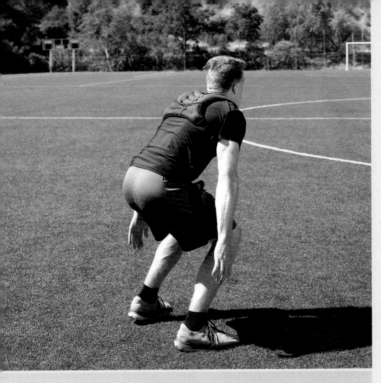

Additional instruction for
JUMP SQUATS WITH WEIGHT

▶ Use 5–10% of body weight, in the form of a weight vest or a dumbbell held in each hand.

▶ If using dumbbells, your arms should remain at your sides throughout the exercise.

▶ By adding weight (with a weight vest or dumbbells), you develop the type of force capacity required for the first-steps acceleration. Plus, research shows that weighted jump squats increase vertical jump height—important in sports like football and basketball.

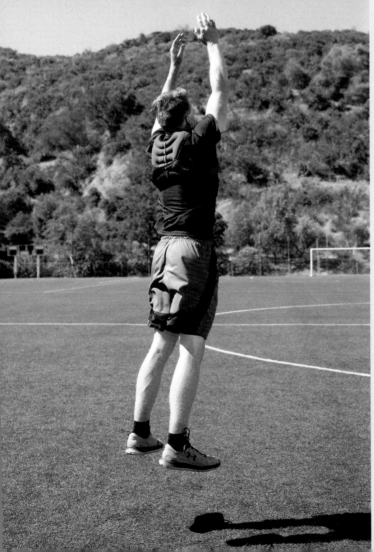

WALKING LUNGES

Walking lunges strengthen your full kinetic chain and pretty much every other muscle you use when running. Adding resistance with a weight vest or dumbbells increases the vertical force you'll need to generate with each step. This exercise is a good fit for acceleration, maximum velocity, and strength training—and it's great for injury prevention, too.

176

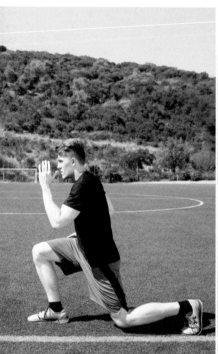 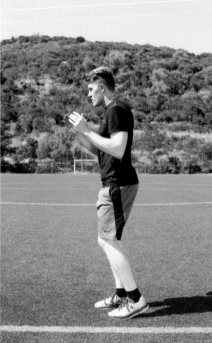 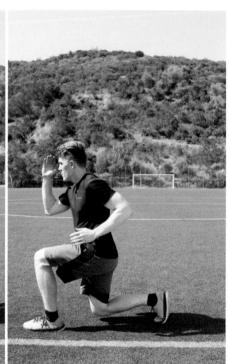

WORKOUT   **10–20 lunges (total for both legs)**

▸ Stand with your feet hip-width apart, toes forward.

▸ Step forward, lowering your hips and bending your front knee until your front thigh is parallel to the ground. Keep your hands on your hips or mimic sprinting arm motion, keeping your elbows at approximately 90°.

▸ Rise as you step forward. Pause for a moment as you reach a standing position in order to assure stability, and then step into a new lunge with the opposite leg.

▸ Alternate feet for the remainder of the repetition.

COACH'S 2 CENTS

When stepping forward into a lunge, your lunge (forward) knee should never extend beyond the toes of your same-side foot.

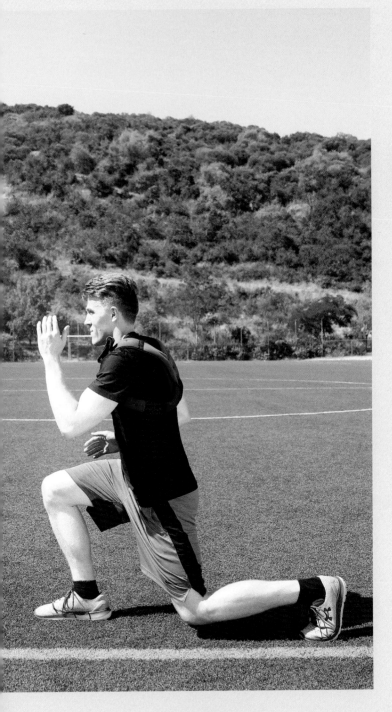

Additional instruction for
ADDING A WEIGHT VEST OR DUMBBELLS

▶ Strap the weight vest on or hold equal-weight dumbbells in each hand with arms extended toward the ground.

▶ If you struggle with form and/or balance, remove the weight and finish the exercise using only body weight.

ANKLE POPPERS

Ankle stiffness is a key to both acceleration and maximum velocity. As sprint expert J. B. Morin says, running without stiff ankles is like driving a car with flat tires. This is especially true during maximum velocity, when you'll need to maintain ankle stability for dozens of high-impact steps. Ankle poppers help you develop the endurance required for the long sprint.

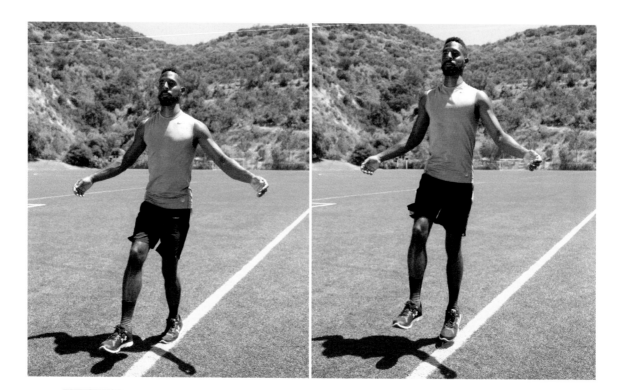

WORKOUT   **2–3 reps of 15 seconds for each leg**

▸ Balance on your left leg with your right leg lifted in front of you. Keep your left knee slightly bent and your arms at your sides for balance.

▸ Hop rapidly up and down on your left foot for 15 seconds.

▸ Switch feet, and hop rapidly up and down on your right foot for 15 seconds.

COACH'S 2 CENTS

The goal isn't to hop as high as you can; it's to hop as quickly as you can.

WEIGHTED ANKLE POPPERS

Weighted ankle poppers, like the bodyweight version of the exercise, stiffen your ankles and develop speed endurance, plus they help you to create lateral force. By hopping back and forth, you also add a component of agility to the exercise—the better to execute changes of direction. Finally, extra weight adds to the vertical force both absorbed and generated during each pop, mimicking the increased force you'll need to manage at top-end speed.

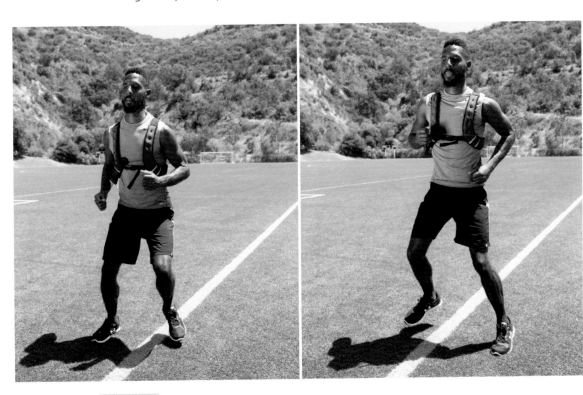

WORKOUT   **2–3 sets of 30–60 seconds each**

▶ Wear a weight vest or hold light (5–10-lb.) dumbbells in each hand.

▶ Jump back and forth from one foot to the other, over a line, while maintaining a slight bend in the knees. Don't move forward; the goal is lateral and vertical motion.

COACH'S 2 CENTS

Perform quick movements, but—in order to avoid increased injury risk from the added weight—focus on keeping your form under control.

DOUBLE-LEG HOPS

The Double-Leg Hop is the poor man's Depth Jump. If you don't have a plyo box or prop swap, you can make do with your own two legs. Instead of dropping from a plyo box, you'll use a countermovement jump to leap to a similar "starting" height. When you land your jump, your legs undergo a strong stretch-shortening cycle and store elastic energy, leading to a powerful rebound jump. You'll train your nervous system for an explosive elastic recoil action.

180

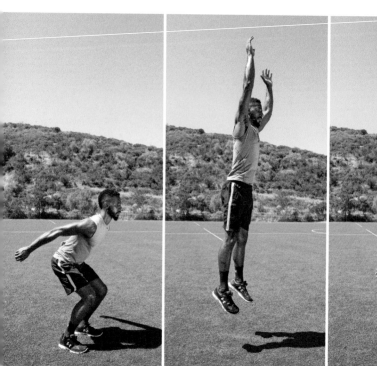
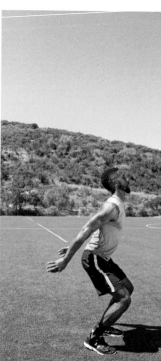
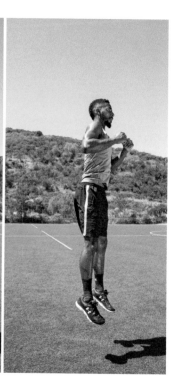

WORKOUT **3–5 reps**

▸ With feet hip-width apart and toes pointed slightly outward, bend your knees to drop into a squat, swinging your arms behind you.

▸ Jump straight up as high as you can.

▸ Land on both feet, letting your knees bend to absorb the force. Swing your arms behind your body as you land.

▸ Spring straight up again, swinging your arms to aid momentum.

COACH'S 2 CENTS

It's the second jump that's key. The first jump is just to get air. The second jump is the "plyometric" part of the exercise—so explode!

SINGLE-LEG HOPS

Once you've mastered the double-leg hop, it's time to try the single-leg version. You'll still be training for a stronger stretch-shortening cycle, minimum transition time between eccentric and concentric contractions, and strong elastic recoil—it's just that this version is a little harder . . . if you guessed twice as hard, you've earned a gold star.

181

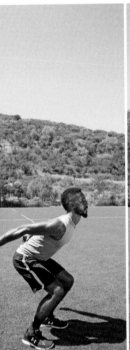
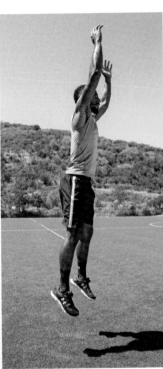
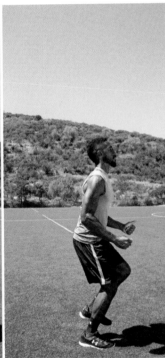
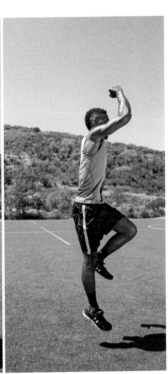

WORKOUT 2-3 reps with each leg (4-6 reps total)

▶ With feet hip-width apart and toes pointed slightly outward, bend your knees to drop into a squat and swing your arms behind you. Jump straight up as high as you can.

▶ Land on your right foot, letting your knee bend to absorb the force.

▶ Bend your left leg behind you, foot off the ground, and spring straight up again. Your arm movement should mimic running form (i.e., right arm and left leg swing forward in sync).

▶ Perform the jump using your left leg.

COACH'S 2 CENTS

Be prepared to see far less vertical height on your single-leg jump than you did for your double-leg jump. This is expected. You're a two-piston engine running on one piston.

STRIDES (90%)

You don't have to run 100 percent effort to improve your top-end speed—90 percent effort will do the trick. Plus, you'll steer clear of nervous system overload and injuries.

182

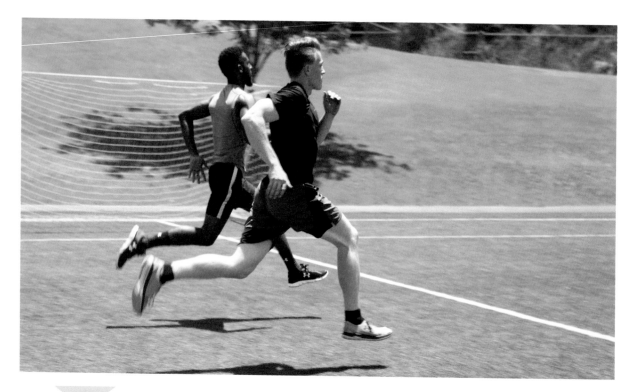

WORKOUT **4–8 reps of 40–50 yards**

▸ Use either a standing start or build into your strides with a few yards of jogging.

▸ Accelerate to approximately 90% of your top-end speed.

▸ Hold it until your reach the 40- or 50-yard mark.

COACH'S 2 CENTS

The entire stride is 40–50 yards, including acceleration and 90%-effort running, so don't wait until you hit 90% speed to start measuring the distance.

GASSERS 30/30

This is a great finishing exercise—mostly because you're too gassed to keep exercising once you're finished. Most exercises and drills in the SpeedRunner schedules rely upon the anaerobic phosphagen system for energy. Gassers draw heavily on your anaerobic glycolysis and aerobic systems. The immediate result is greater fatigue. The long-term result is better speed endurance.

183

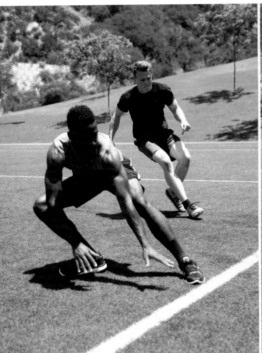
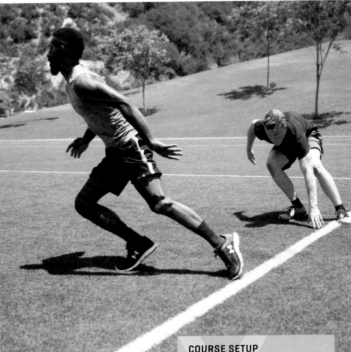

WORKOUT   **2–8 reps (120 yards total per rep)**

▸ Begin from a standing start on the start line.

▸ Run at 90% maximum speed for 30 yards to the second line. Touch down on the line, then reverse direction. Run 30 yards to the start line, touch down, and reverse direction.

▸ Run once more down and back, touching down at the second line again.

▸ Finish at the start line—a total of four lengths of the 30-yard course and 3 touch downs.

▸ Rest for 2–3 minutes, then repeat.

COURSE SETUP
Use lines on the field, cones, or prop swaps to mark two lines (or objects) separated by 30 yards.

COACH'S 2 CENTS

Focus on seamless change-of-direction transitions after each touch down. And limit yourself to 90% max velocity, or you'll fade before the workout is done, and you'll incur more fatigue than you can recover from by the next day.

METRICS TESTING

40-YARD DASH

The 40-Yard Dash is one of the most popular tests for measuring acceleration and speed, no matter the sport. For most speedsters, 40 yards provides enough distance to churn through all phases of acceleration and reach maximum velocity. SpeedRunner training can improve your 40-yard performance up to 10 percent.

186

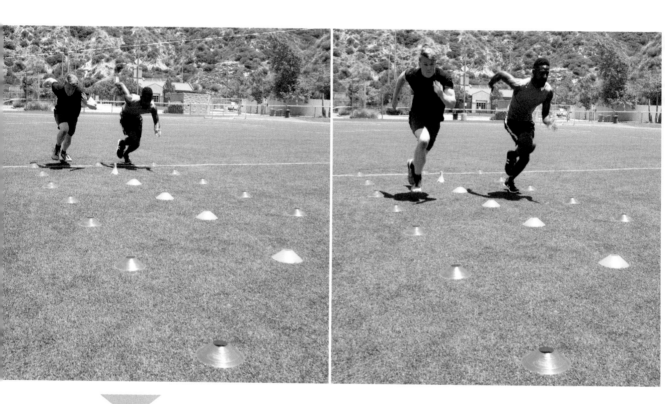

WORKOUT   1–2 reps (when testing, take best of 2 times)

▸ Take a 3-point stance (see page 125), with your down hand immediately behind the start line. If you haven't learned a 3-point stance, a standing start is okay.

▸ On command, sprint 40 yards in a straight line.

COACH'S 2 CENTS

This is an all-out effort from the start. Don't pace yourself. Explode.

STANDING BROAD JUMP

The Standing Broad Jump is a great test of your ability to produce both horizontal and vertical force. A 2015 study found "significant correlations" between the length of athletes' standing broad jumps and their times at 10, 30, and 100 meters—in other words, jumping performance correlated to every phase of sprinting from initial acceleration to maximum velocity and including the final meters of deceleration.

187

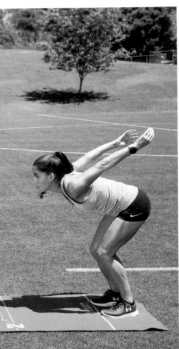
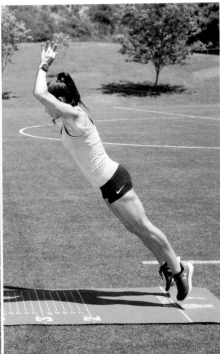
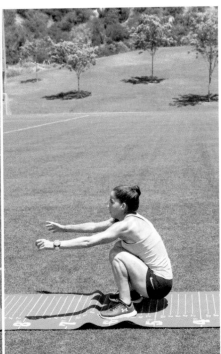

WORKOUT   **1–2 reps (when testing, take best of 2 times)**

▸ Stand at the start (jump) line with feet hip-to-shoulder-width apart.

▸ Quickly squat, swinging your arms behind you, then spring forward while swinging your arms in front of your body.

▸ Land on both feet and stick your landing—if you fall forward or backward, the jump doesn't count.

▸ Measure your distance from the back of the heel that's closest to the start line.

COACH'S 2 CENTS

Practice this jump a few times before testing. Just as there's a perfect arc for throwing a ball to ensure the greatest distance, there's a perfect angle for you to launch yourself into the air.

20-YARD SHUTTLE

The 20-Yard Shuttle tests explosiveness (first steps acceleration), agility, lateral quickness, change-of-direction ability, balance, and coordination. This exercise is featured at the NFL combine and is regularly included in skills testing for soccer, baseball, and hockey, among other sports.

188

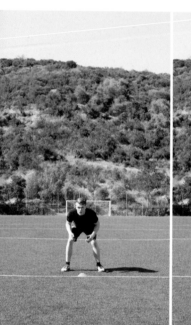 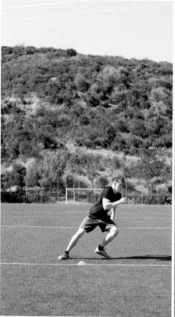 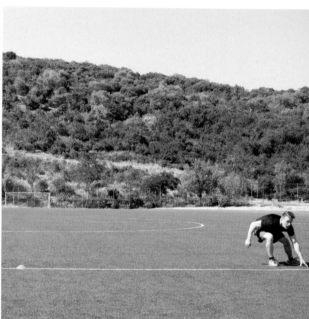

WORKOUT 1–2 reps (when testing, take best of two times)

▸ Start in either a 3-point stance (down hand immediately behind the center cone) or from a standing position with feet shoulder-width apart, knees bent, and arms at your sides.

▸ On command, sprint 5 yards from the center cone to the right or left cone, depending on predetermined direction. Touch the ground immediately beyond the cone with the same-side hand as the direction you sprinted.

▸ Reverse direction, sprinting 10 yards to the opposite end-cone. Touch the ground immediately beyond the cone with your other hand.

▸ Reverse direction again, sprinting 5 yards. The center cone is the finish line.

COACH'S 2 CENTS

At the NFL combine, players must start from a modified 3-point stance (both feet parallel) and sprint to the right-side cone first. For SpeedRunner, you'll practice both directions, as your ultimate goal is better all-around agility, not an NFL-standard test result. When starting this drill, make your first step a crossover step—pivot off the foot nearest your first target cone and take your first step with your opposite leg, crossing over your pivot-foot leg.

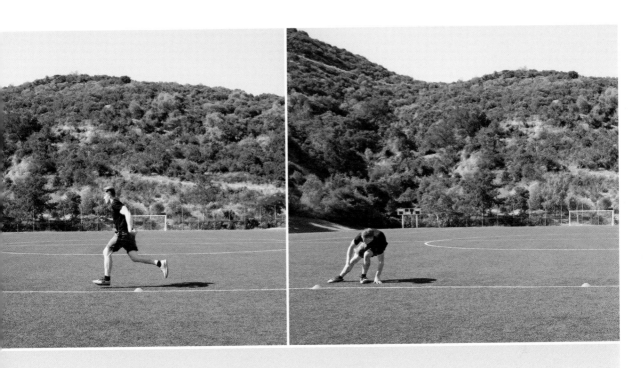

COURSE SETUP
Place 3 cones (or prop swaps) 5 yards apart on a single line (i.e., 10 yards total).

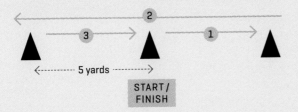

5 yards

START / FINISH

3-CONE DRILL

Like the 20-Yard Shuttle, this drill tests acceleration, explosiveness, agility, change-of-direction ability, balance, and coordination. Research has found that the results of this test and the 20-Yard Shuttle correlate almost perfectly, which means they're probably testing similar abilities. If you've completed the full range of SpeedRunner training, you should do well in both.

190

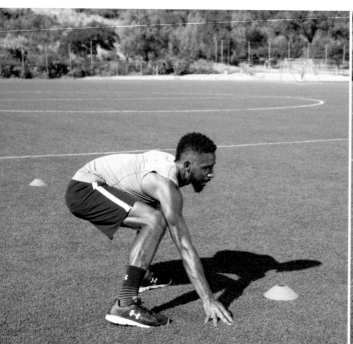 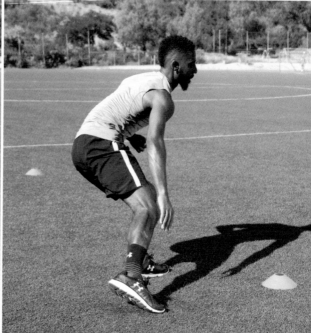

WORKOUT 1–2 reps (when testing, take best of 2 times)

▸ Begin in a 3-point stance, with your down hand behind the start-line cone.

▸ On command, sprint 5 yards to cone 2 and touch the ground immediately beyond it.

▸ Reverse direction, sprinting back to cone 1 and touching the ground beyond it.

▸ Reverse direction again, sprinting back toward cone 2.

▸ Sprint around the outside of cone 2, then weave to the inside of cone 3.

▸ Cut around cone 3 and sprint back toward cone 2.

▸ Cut around the outside of cone 2 and sprint past cone 1—your finish line.

COACH'S 2 CENTS

At the NFL combine, players start in a 3-point stance, then touch down at cone 2 with their right hand, come back to cone 1 and touch down with their right hand again, then sprint back to cone 2 and turn 90° right, before weaving underneath cone 3 and then sprinting back around cone 2 to the finish. For SpeedRunner, use either hand for touching down and alternate direction at cone 2; alternating directions offers better agility training.

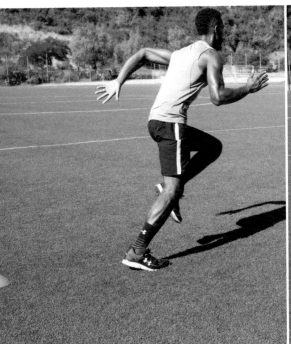 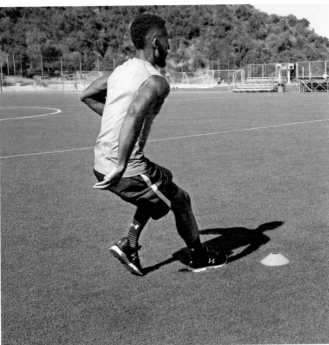

COURSE SETUP

Use 3 cones (or prop swaps), set up in an "L" pattern (90° angle), with the cones 5 yards apart. Then add 1 more cone, creating an "L" pattern in the opposite direction.

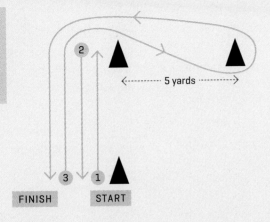

SPEEDRUNNER WORKOUTS

STRENGTH TRAINING

AIR SQUATS

Squats activate your glutes and work your quadriceps. The push you get from knee extension (quadriceps contraction) is vital for the first 5 yards of acceleration. A 2015 study found that squats plus repeated sprint training [e.g., the Strides (90%) exercise] improved sprint performance by over 2%, while a 2016 study concluded that quarter squats worked better than half and full squats for improving speed.

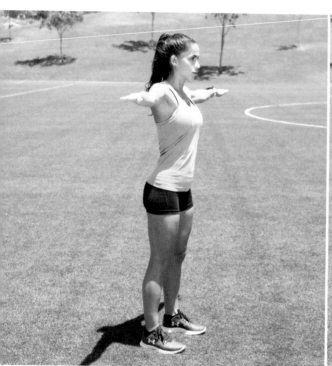 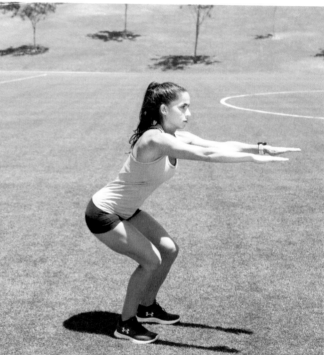

WORKOUT   **2–3 sets of 5–10 reps**

▸ Stand with your feet hip-width apart, toes pointed slightly out, and arms extended straight out from your shoulders.

▸ Squat by pushing your hips back and bending your knees. As you squat, swing your arms forward along a horizontal plane until they're extended in front of your shoulders. Pause when your thighs are near-parallel or parallel to the ground—a quarter squat for maximum velocity training and half squat for acceleration.

▸ Return to your start position and repeat.

COACH'S 2 CENTS

You don't have to squat so low that your thighs are parallel to the ground. While a lower squat will help acceleration, a quarter squat gives you more bang for your maximum velocity buck.

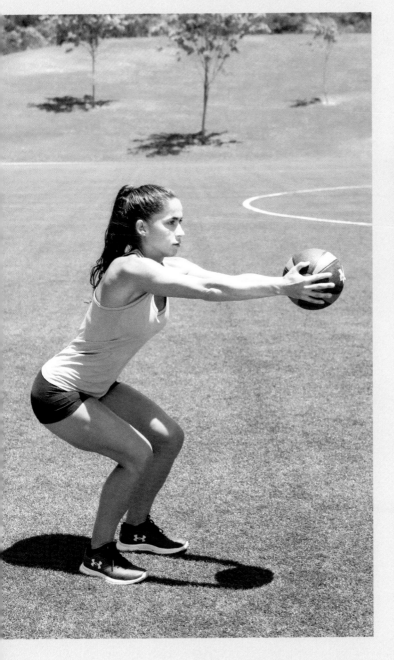

Additional instruction
WITH MEDBALL

▶ To add balance and increase difficulty, begin with a medball held in front of you, arms extended.

▶ Perform your air squat while continuing to hold the medball in front of you.

BEAR CRAWL

This exercise takes many of us back to childhood, when we bear crawled just for the fun of it. Now that you're older, bear crawling might not be as much fun, but it's a perfect full-body strengthening exercise. Done correctly, you'll develop lower-back stability and get a terrific core workout.

196

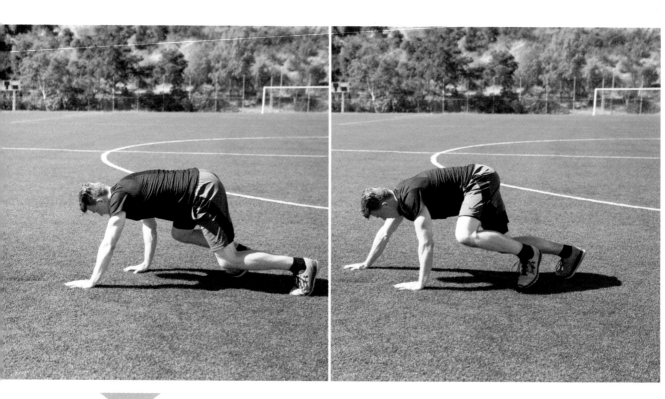

WORKOUT 1–2 sets of 10–30 yards or 10 yards forward + 10 yards backward

▶ Begin on all fours—hands beneath shoulders, knees beneath hips, spine straight. Lift your knees a few inches off the ground, keeping your weight on your toes and balls of your feet.

▶ Move your left hand and right foot forward simultaneously. Set them down, and repeat the action with your right hand and left foot. Avoid swiveling sideways as you crawl—a common beginner's mistake.

▶ Crawl straight ahead, or for variation, crawl forward 10 yards, then reverse direction and crawl backward for an equal distance.

COACH'S 2 CENTS

Keep head, back, and hips in a straight and level line throughout the exercise. Don't stick your butt up in the air—you should be able to balance a glass of water on your back while performing this exercise. Less-fit athletes might require a slightly wider stance with their hands and knees.

CRAB WALK

This one is tougher than it looks. So tough, in fact, that you have permission, right out of the gate, to get out of sync—wrong hand to foot, lifting one limb at a time, etc.— as you perform it. Crab walking strengthens your shoulders, triceps, core, glutes, and hamstrings. As you strive to keep full-body muscle balance, this is a key exercise.

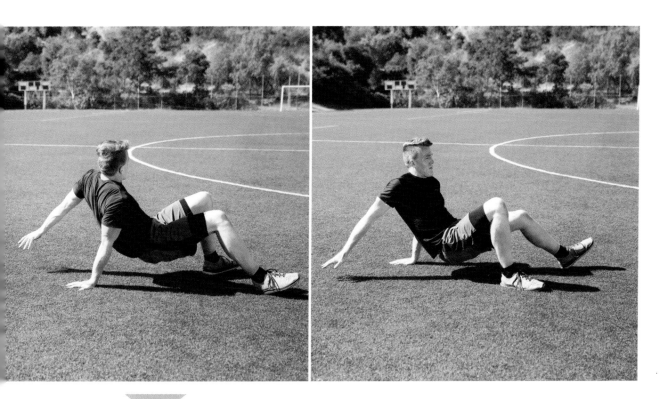

WORKOUT   **1–2 sets of 10–20 yards**

▶ Begin in a supine position (face up), while resting on your hands and heels. Hands should be shoulder-width apart, heels hip-width apart. Your butt should clear the ground by only a few inches (i.e., don't create an abdominal bridge). Angle your fingers away from your body, or find a position that reduces strain on your wrists.

▶ Lift your right hand and left foot and move in the direction that lies behind your head.

▶ Put your hand and foot down, and then move your left hand and right foot.

COACH'S 2 CENTS

This exercise can be hard on the wrists, so some athletes prefer to perform the crab walk on their fingertips. Don't worry if your butt droops— it's supposed to. And don't worry if you get out of sync. You'll still get the work.

BIRD DOGS

This is a great exercise for stabilizing the muscles that control your spine, developing general core strength, and preventing lower back stress and abdominal stitches.

198

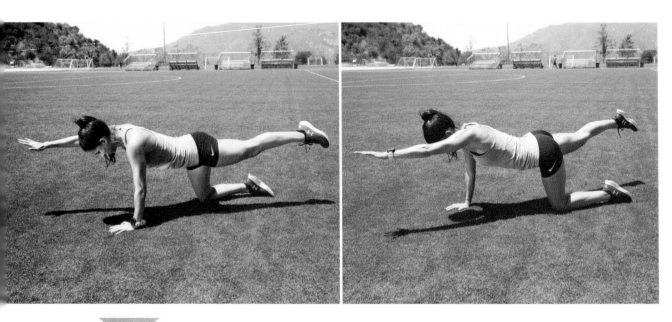

WORKOUT 1–2 sets of 5–10 reps, each side, alternating sides (10–20 reps total)

▸ Begin on all fours—hands beneath shoulders, knees beneath hips, spine straight. Keep your eyes focused on the ground.

▸ Simultaneously lift your right arm and left leg, extending your arm straight ahead and extending your leg backward. Hold for 1–2 seconds, then return to start position.

▸ Perform the same movement with the left arm and right leg.

FIRE HYDRANT

This is a great exercise for strengthening your hip abductor muscles. It got its name exactly the way you think it got its name. If you're having trouble with form, just take your dog for a walk and observe.

199

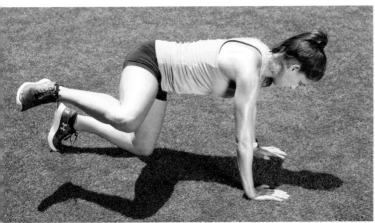

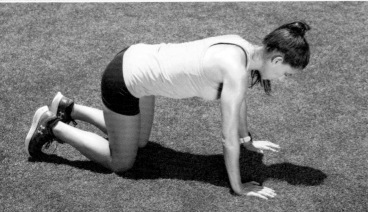

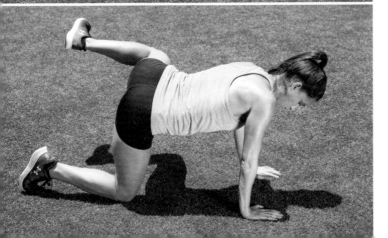

WORKOUT **1–2 sets of 5–10 reps each side (10–20 reps total)**

▶ Begin on all fours—hands beneath shoulders, knees beneath hips, spine straight.

▶ Lift your right leg to the side, maintaining a 90° angle at the knee. Keep lifting until your thigh is parallel to the ground. Control your leg as you return to the start position.

▶ Repeat until you've finished your reps with one leg.

▶ Switch to the other leg and do all reps for that leg.

COACH'S 2 CENTS

Lift your thighs laterally from your hips, not forward or backward.

LEG LIFTS

Leg Lifts strengthen your abs and hip flexors, aiding core stability and knee lift.
By controlling the descent of your legs, you strengthen your hip flexors eccentrically—
essential for powering the strong hip flexor stretch reflex that ends stance phase and
kicks off swing phase.

200

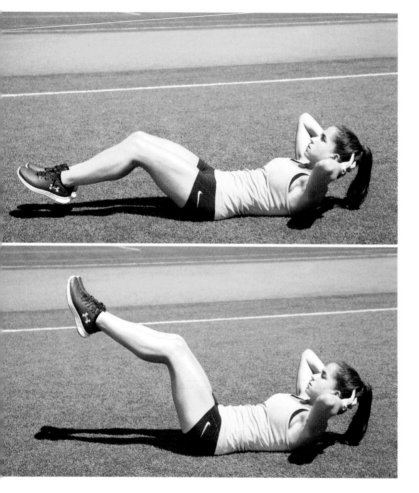

WORKOUT   **1 set of 15–50 reps**

▶ Lie on your back with your
knees slightly bent. Lift your
head, linking hands behind
your head for support.

▶ Keeping your torso stable,
lift your legs to 45° while
maintaining the bend at the
knees.

▶ Don't hold the position—
instead, lower your legs at
a controlled (not slow) rate.

▶ When your heels are within
an inch or two of the ground
(i.e., before they touch down),
reverse direction for your
next rep.

COACH'S 2 CENTS

Throughout the exercise, maintain
a consistent bend at your knees
that mimics the flexion you
experience during stance phase
while running. For most athletes,
this translates to 15–45° of flexion.

MARCHING BRIDGE

Not only is this a good exercise for strengthening your lower back, glutes, and hamstrings, it's also a great way to prevent or reduce lower-back pain.

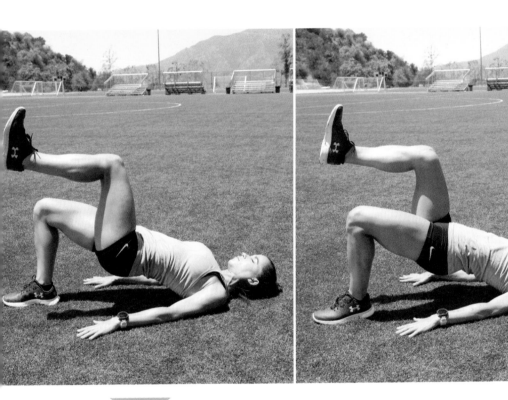

WORKOUT **1–2 sets of 5–10 reps with each leg (10–20 reps total)**

▸ Lie on the ground in a supine (face up) position. Extend your arms to your sides, with your feet hip-width apart, soles of your feet on the ground.

▸ Lift your hips to form a straight line from your knees to your shoulders.

▸ Raise one leg at a time, keeping about a 90° angle at the knee, marching your knees toward your chest.

COACH'S 2 CENTS

Keep your foot dorsiflexed (i.e., lifted toward your shin).

NORDIC CURLS

This exercise is not only a top hamstring injury-prevention exercise (see "Hammy Time," page 61), it's also a demanding eccentric hamstring-strengthening exercise—preparing you for late stance phase, when your hamstrings endure loads of 8–10 times your body weight. The only drawback to Nordic Curls is the lack of movement in the hip joint (the hamstrings flex the knee joint and extend the hip joint), but if you pair these with single-leg deadlifts, you'll have your hamstrings covered.

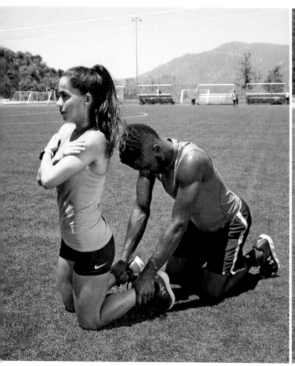 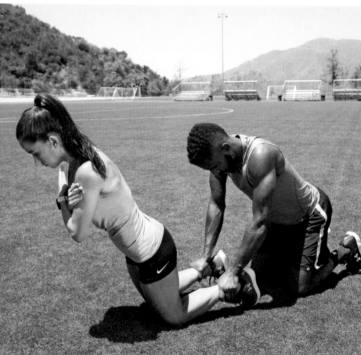

WORKOUT 1–2 sets of 2–10 reps

▸ Kneel, with arms crossed and held against your chest. You'll need either a partner to pin your ankles or something to hold them in place (e.g., hook them beneath a bedframe).

▸ Bend forward from the knees, slowly lowering yourself to the ground. Keep a straight line from your spine through your knees. If you start to fall, use your hands to stop your descent.

▸ Use your arms to thrust yourself back up to the starting position (i.e., don't work this exercise in reverse!).

COACH'S 2 CENTS

Don't worry if you can't hold yourself up very well at first. Some athletes find they can't hold themselves at all—and are lucky to get their hands out in time to avoid a bloody nose. It can take your nervous system a few sessions to master control of your hamstrings. After a couple sessions, you'll feel in control.

MOUNTAIN CLIMBERS

This is primarily a powerful hip flexor exercise, but you'll also target core, shoulder, and arm strength. The key to this exercise is keeping a level plane from your back through your hips—don't let your hips bob up and down during reps.

203

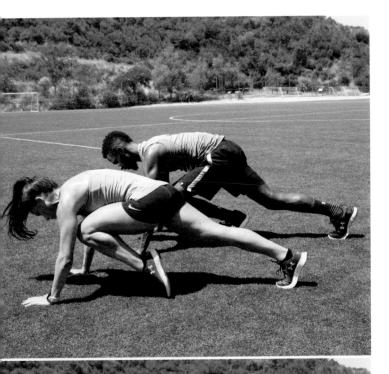

WORKOUT 2–3 sets of 20–30 seconds

▶ Start from the top of a push-up position, arms extended beneath shoulders.

▶ Drive your right knee forward, toward your chest.

▶ Quickly reverse your right knee, thrusting it backward, while simultaneously driving your left knee forward.

▶ Don't pause between reps— your legs are like pistons in a fast-moving engine.

COACH'S 2 CENTS

You might want your hands a little wider than push-up position—that's perfectly acceptable. Stay balanced on the toes of your extended limb throughout the exercise.

PLANK

Ah yes, the classic core-targeting exercise. Sometimes you just can't improve on the original. You'll target spinal stabilization while developing a strong and powerful core and torso.

204

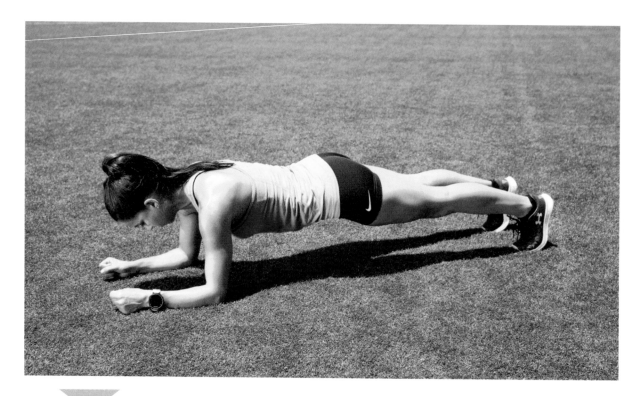

WORKOUT   **1–2 sets of 30 seconds**

▶ Start in a plank position: rest on elbows and toes, with elbows beneath shoulders at a 90° angle and ensuring a straight line from your head to your heels.

▶ Hold, squeezing your glutes and tightening your abdominals to maintain the position.

COACH'S 2 CENTS

It's easy to let your mind wander, your back sway, and your butt sag during planks—don't.

PLANK ROTATIONS

This variation on a traditional Plank adds extra strengthening for your shoulders and upper back, while still producing all the great core strengthening you've come to expect from the original. You'll also train your nervous system to maintain spinal stability while your upper torso is in motion.

205

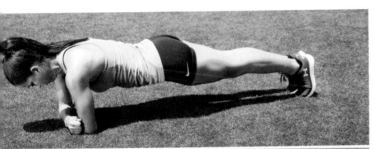

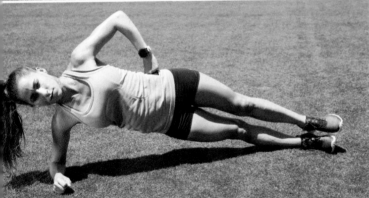

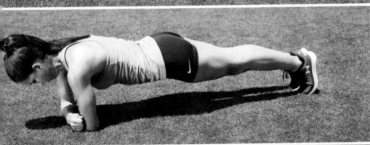

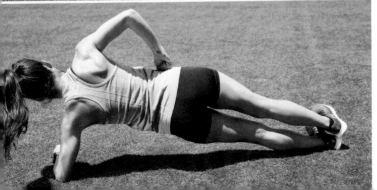

WORKOUT 1–2 sets of 5–15 reps on each side

▸ Start in a modified push-up position—face down, resting on elbows and toes, spine straight from your head through your heels. Position your forearms horizontally beneath your shoulders, directly parallel to each other.

▸ Rotate onto your right elbow, keeping a straight line from your shoulder through the elbow. Place your left hand on your hip and keep your spine straight.

▸ Return to your start position.

▸ Rotate onto your left elbow.

▸ Alternate sides until you've completed your repetitions.

COACH'S 2 CENTS

Maintain a controlled rhythm—not fast, not slow—while performing this exercise. The object is to develop rotational stability that will aid speed and agility.

SIDE LEG LIFTS

This straightforward exercise strengthens your hip abductors. While you won't get the dynamic abductor workout of Side Steps (Quick)—or the sprint/agility-specific benefits of Weight Sled Crossovers, Monster Walks, or Side Steps with Resistance Band— Side Leg Lifts will help with the initial strengthening of your abductors that makes those more intense exercises possible.

206

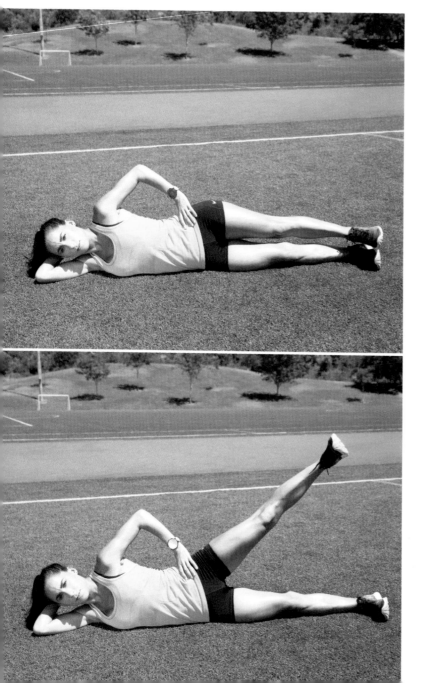

WORKOUT **1–2 sets of 10–15 reps with each leg**

▶ Lie on your right side, legs stacked, right arm folded beneath your head for a pillow. Rest your left hand on your hip. Maintain a straight line through your head, spine, and hips.

▶ Lift your left leg in a smooth, controlled motion to 45°.

▶ Use an equally controlled motion to return to your start position.

▶ Finish your left leg reps, then switch to your right leg.

SINGLE-LEG SQUAT

Single-Leg Squats add resistance to bodyweight squats (i.e., by working with only one leg, you double the load), and also target balance and stability. You'll work your quads, glutes, and hamstrings, as well as your abductors, which keep your hips on a level plane. Many athletes use a prop (e.g., a chair or bench) the first few times they perform this exercise.

207

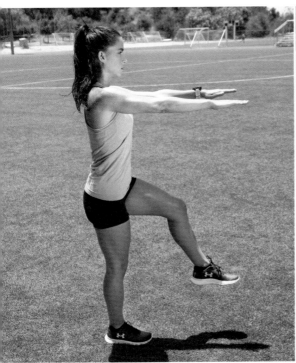 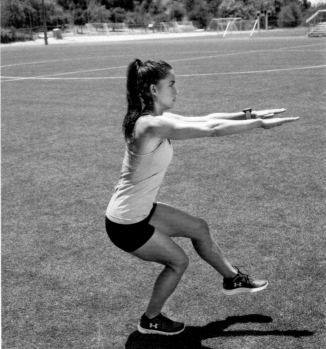

WORKOUT 1-2 sets of 5-10 reps with each leg

▸ Begin from a standing position, feet hip-width apart, with arms straight out in front of you.

▸ Lift your left leg, with the thigh at 45° and the knee bent. Your right leg should be slightly bent at the knee (for balance). Lower yourself into a squat—one-quarter to one-half-squat, no deeper.

▸ Press down on your heel as you return to your start position.

▸ Finish all reps with your right leg, then switch legs.

Additional instruction
FROM A SEATED POSITION

▸ Sit on a chair (or other prop), arms extended from your shoulders.

▸ Start with your right foot on the ground, your left thigh angled at 45°.

▸ Press down on your foot and stand up, then slowly sit back down.

SINGLE-LEG DEADLIFT

Single-Leg Deadlifts, which work the hamstrings eccentrically, are the perfect companion exercise to Nordic Curls. While Nordic Curls incorporate movement at the knee joint, Single-Leg Deadlifts focus on movement at the hip joint (your hamstrings both flex the knee and extend the hip). Together, these exercises give your hamstrings the maximum eccentric workout. Single-Leg Deadlifts also mimic your leg's stance-phase posture during sprinting.

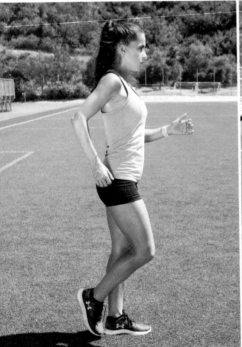
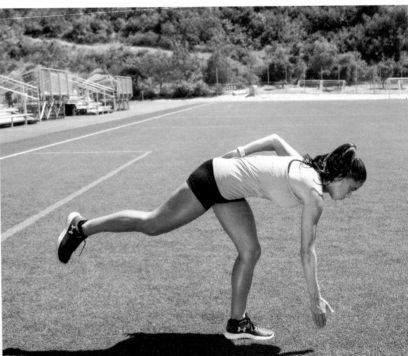

▼ **WORKOUT**   **1–2 sets of 5–10 reps for each leg**

▶ Stand with feet hip-width apart.

▶ Lift your right foot off the ground by bending your knee; your left knee should also have a slight bend.

▶ Bend forward from your hips, reaching your right hand toward the ground. Simultaneously, lift and extend your right leg behind you. Maintain a slight bend in both knees.

▶ Return to your start position, finish your reps with your right leg down, and then switch legs.

COACH'S 2 CENTS

If support is needed, you can rest one hand on a chair or other object. Use the same-side hand as your down leg for this purpose. Don't do this exercise with straight legs—that defeats the purpose. You're trying to strengthen your hamstring eccentrically while mimicking stance-phase posture.

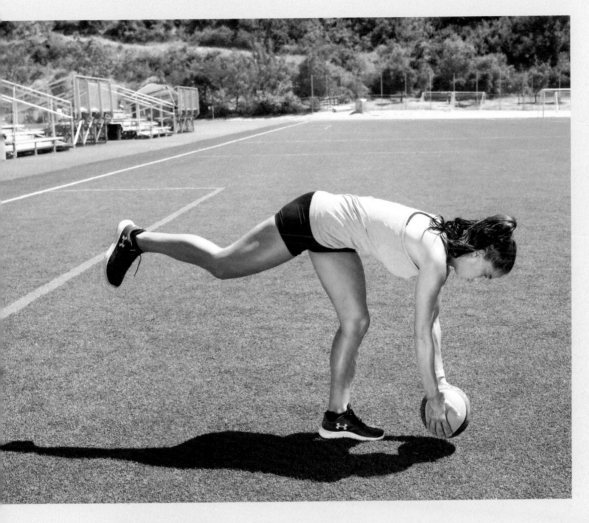

Additional instruction
WITH MEDBALL OR DUMBBELL

▶ **Medball:** Start with the medball in front of your
chest. Lower it to the ground, fully extending
your arms beneath your shoulders.

▶ **Dumbbell:** Start with the weight held at your side
(on the same side as your lifted leg), and then lower
the dumbbell to the ground, extending the opposite
hand behind/above your hip for balance.

SUPERMAN OR SUPERWOMAN PLANK

This variation combines core, shoulder, arm, and back strengthening with an incredible challenge to your balance and proprioception skills. You'll want to master the Plank and Bird Dogs before working up to this exercise.

210

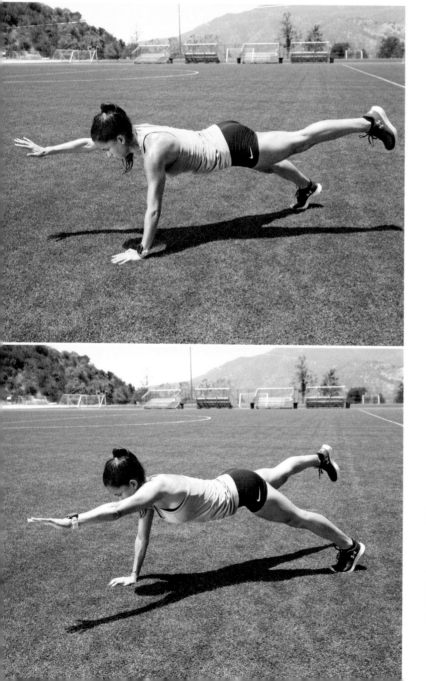

WORKOUT   **1–2 sets of 5–10 reps of 2–3 seconds for each side**

▶ Begin at the top of the push-up position. Simultaneously lift your right arm and left leg, extending both, keeping a level plane from extended arm through extended leg.

▶ Hold for 2–3 seconds.

▶ Return to your start position.

▶ Repeat the above steps for your left arm and right leg. Alternate until all reps are completed.

COACH'S 2 CENTS

Balance is key. If you start to lose your balance, shorten your reps. If you can't keep your balance at all, substitute Bird Dogs (page 198).

V-UPS

With V-Ups, you'll target your core muscles with a more intense workout than traditional sit-ups. If regular V-Up intensity isn't enough, add a medball to the mix.

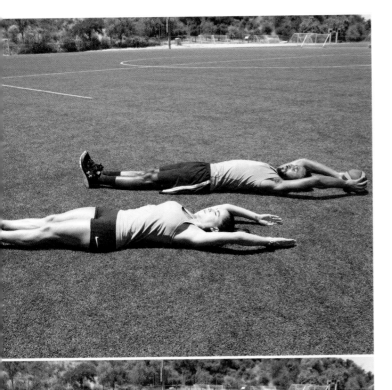

1–2 sets of 5–10 reps

▶ Lie on your back, with arms stretched over your head, and legs straight and flat on the ground.

▶ Simultaneously lift arms and legs off the ground, keeping all limbs straight. Touch your toes to your hands (or as close as you are able).

▶ Return to your start position.

Additional instruction for
USING A MEDBALL

▶ Hold the medball in your hands (or, for advanced athletes, between your feet).

▶ Perform the exercise exactly as you did without the medball.

WINDSHIELD WIPERS

Windshield Wipers target your full range of abdominal muscles and improve rotational stability.

212

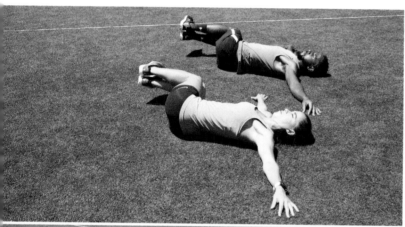

1–2 sets of 8–10 reps for each side

▸ Lie in a supine (face up) position, with arms extended straight out from your shoulders.

▸ Lift your legs—90° angle at your hips and 90° angle at your knees.

▸ Rotate your legs to the right side, keeping your legs together and your feet dorsiflexed (i.e., lifted toward your shin). Rotate until you're almost touching the ground— but don't touch.

▸ Return to your start position, then repeat while rotating to the left side.

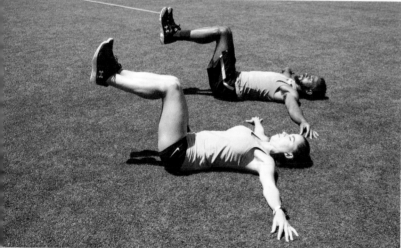

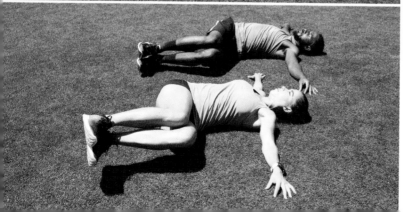

COACH'S 2 CENTS

Make sure that your upper back maintains contact with the ground throughout your rotation in both directions.

KNEELING PARTNER MEDBALL TWIST

This is a terrific two-person exercise. You'll target your entire core musculature, with a special emphasis on your obliques. Trunk rotation is essential in most team sports.

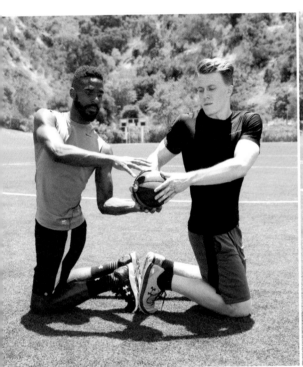 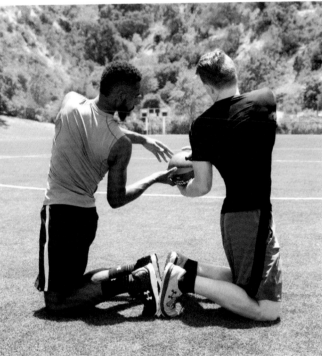

WORKOUT 1 rep (continuously passing the medball) each direction (2 reps total), 30–60 seconds each

▶ Kneel facing away from your partner, with the soles of your shoes touching your partner's soles. Maintain a straight line from your head through your knees. Hold the medball in front of your chest, a slight bend at your elbows.

▶ Twist right to pass the medball to your partner, who twists left to receive it. Your partner then twists right to hand the medball back to you on the opposite side.

▶ Rest for up to a minute, then repeat in the opposite direction.

COACH'S 2 CENTS

Keep your abs tight and the motion fluid throughout the exercise. If you don't have a partner, do the exercise solo: From a kneeling position, twist in one direction while holding the medball, stopping when you reach the limit to your range of motion (don't rotate to the point of discomfort), then reverse direction and perform the same movement to the opposite side.

HIP THRUST

Want great hip extension? The Hip Thrust can help you achieve it. Bret Contreras, known as The Glute Guy, has long championed this exercise for sprinters. He points out that Hip Thrusts activate the glutes to 119 percent maximum voluntary contraction, while lunges register a paltry 30 percent. In fact, Hip Thrusts will activate your glutes more than any other bodyweight exercise. They're also key to developing hip hyperextension strength—a must for speedsters.

214

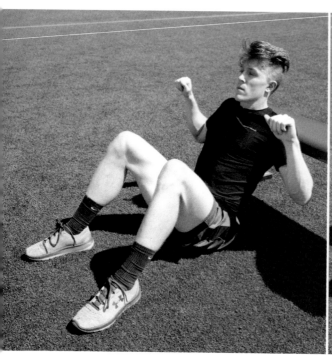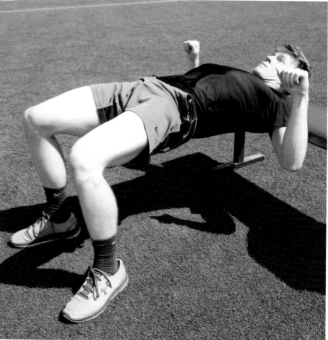

WORKOUT 1–2 sets of 3–5 reps to start, building to 10 reps over a few sessions

▸ Sit on the ground, knees bent, feet flat, and lean your back against a stable bench (or other platform). The edge of the bench should touch the low point of your shoulder blades. Your feet and legs should be angled slightly outward. With a 90° bend at the elbows, hold your arms slightly out from your sides, with your hands curled in front of your chest, as if holding a barbell.

▸ Use your glutes to lift your pelvis off the ground, forming a bridge from your shoulders to your knees— your knees should form a 90° angle; if they don't, adjust foot placement. Lift your pelvis as high as you can.

▸ Don't hold the position; instead, drop back to the start.

▸ Repeat, using a steady rhythm for your reps.

COACH'S 2 CENTS

If you haven't done this exercise before, take it easy the first few times. Glute activation is high, and you'll have a sore butt if you're not careful. Three quick form tips: Push through the heels (not the balls of your feet), rock your pelvis slightly toward your chest while thrusting to ensure full glute activation, and don't let your knees fold inward or outward.

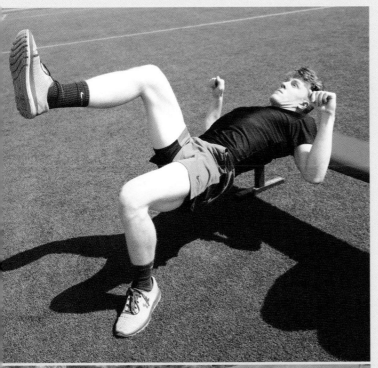

Additional instruction for
SINGLE LEG HIP THRUST

▸ From the same initial hip thrust position, lift one foot a few inches off the ground.

▸ As you hip thrust, lift the elevated leg so that the thigh finishes at a 90° angle to your pelvis, with up to a 90° angle for the elevated knee.

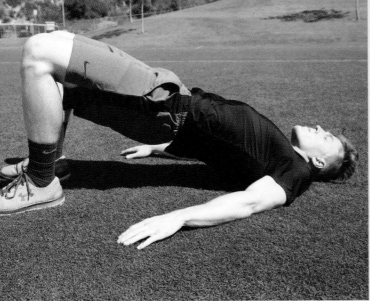

Additional instruction for
SUPINE HIP THRUST

▸ If you don't have a platform, then lie on your back, arms extended out to your sides. Your heels should be positioned close to your glutes.

▸ Use your glutes to lift your pelvis, forming a straight line from your knees to your shoulders.

LUNGE CLOCK

The Lunge Clock requires you to perform bodyweight lunges in multiple directions, building balance and strength for multiple muscle groups (e.g., core, quadriceps, glutes, hamstrings, abductors, and adductors), as well as developing stability in all directions: forward, backward, and lateral.

216

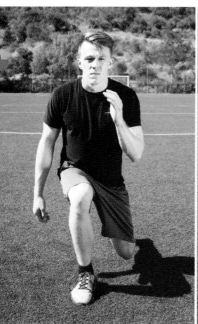
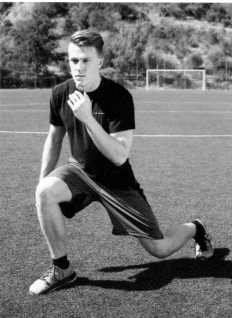
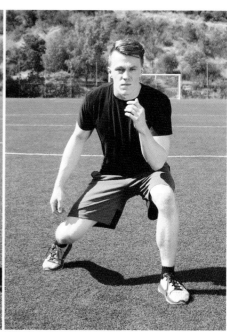

WORKOUT **1 rep clockwise and 1 rep counterclockwise (2 reps total)**

▶ Stand with feet hip-width apart, toes pointed forward, arms at your side.

▶ Step forward with your right leg into a bodyweight lunge. This is the "12 o'clock" position.

▶ Return to your start position, then again with your right leg, lunge forward and slightly to the right, to the 1:30 position.

▶ Return to your start position.

▶ Lunge "around the clock" at the 3:00, 4:30, 6:00 (a backward lunge), 7:30 (switch lunging leg), 9:00, and 10:30.

▶ Rest for 1–2 minutes, then do the exercise in reverse—this time doing the 12 o'clock lunge with your left leg.

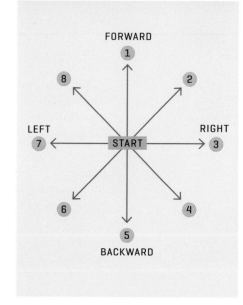

TUG ROPE WITH WEIGHT SLED OR FREE WEIGHT

This full-body exercise works your forearms, biceps, and back, as well as your quadriceps, glutes, hamstrings, and calves—and pretty much works every other muscle along the way, too. If you can find a few people who'd like to engage in an actual, human-on-human tug-of-war, then by all means substitute that for this.

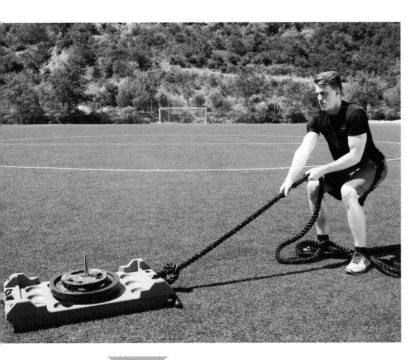

WORKOUT   **1–2 reps of your rope's full length**

- ▶ Load your sled with the desired weight, or attach the rope to free weight (e.g., a weight plate or sand bag).

- ▶ Begin in a partial squat—feet shoulder-width apart, toes pointed slightly outward, shoulders squared forward. Hold the rope in both hands, right hand in front of your left hand.

- ▶ Pull the rope toward your belly with your right hand, while reaching forward with your left hand to grasp the rope. Pull backward with your left hand, releasing the rope with your right hand.

- ▶ Continue this hand-over-hand motion until the weight sled is near your feet—don't pull the sled or weight off the ground.

No-prop alternative:
PULL-UPS

If you don't have a weight sled, you can get a similar upper-body workout from Pull-Ups, although it won't simulate the lower-body work you'll get from Tug Rope.

- ▶ Grab a pull-up bar with your hands shoulder-width or more apart. Hang from the bar while crossing your legs at your ankles and maintaining a slight bend at the knees to relieve stress on your lower back.

- ▶ Pull yourself up until your chin reaches or crests the bar. It's okay if your body angles forward during this exercise, but avoid using body swings to aid the Pull-Up.

- ▶ Return to the start position, then repeat 3–5 times— or more, if fitness allows.

BATTLE ROPES

For a fun, dynamic alternative to traditional upper-body resistance training, nothing beats Battle Ropes. Use 1.5-inch thick rope, in 30-, 40-, or 50-foot lengths—the longer the rope, the greater the resistance. You'll work your shoulders, back, and arms as you create various wave patterns with the rope. But don't expect it to be easy. The first few times, you can expect to develop significant shoulder fatigue within 15–20 seconds.

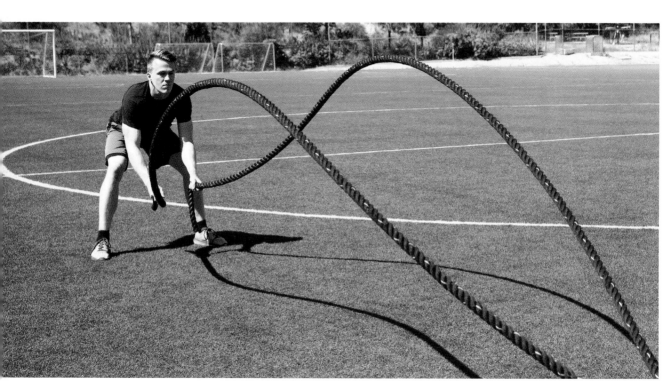

WORKOUT   2–3 sets of 15–30 seconds

▶ Stand with your feet shoulder-width apart, knees bent, rope ends held at shoulder height.

▶ Flick the rope up quickly, then crash down with maximum force to create a wave.

▶ Immediately raise your arms again, to at least head level, and repeat the wave-making motion with your arms.

COACH'S 2 CENTS

As you drive your arms down to create waves, imagine trying to slap the ground with the ropes.

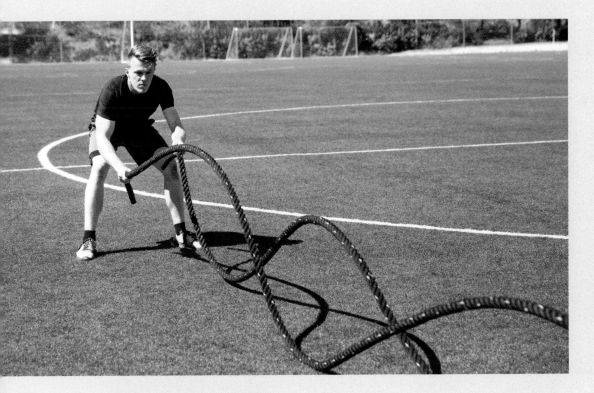

Additional instruction for creating
ALTERNATING WAVES:

▶ To create alternating waves
(i.e., one side peaking while the other
is at the bottom of its cycle), begin
with one hand at head height and
one at waist level.

▶ Create a piston-like motion—
one arm up, one down, then quickly
reverse. This will create smaller,
more frequent waves.

OVERHEAD MEDBALL THROW

This exercise works muscles from head to toe—although "toe to head" is probably a more accurate description, since you'll utilize a transfer of power from your lower to upper body to launch the medball over your head. If you perform this exercise correctly, you'll be shocked at the force you can generate. Just make sure no one's standing within 30–40 yards behind you when you let fly.

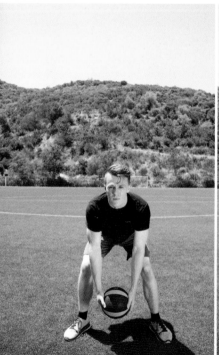 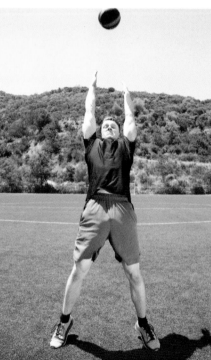 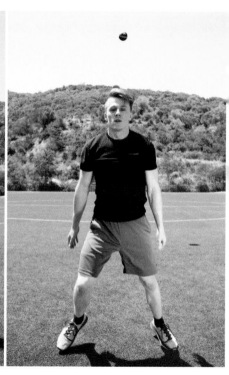

WORKOUT   **3–5 reps**

▸ Stand with your feet shoulder-width apart, toes pointed slightly outward. Hold the medball in front of your chest, elbows at your sides.

▸ Drop into a quarter squat, bringing the medball between your knees.

▸ Explode upward, fully extending your hips and knees as you come up on the balls of your feet, throwing the medball over your head and behind you.

COACH'S 2 CENTS

Focus on throwing the ball both vertically and horizontally (i.e., not just up). Let your body complete its recovery action before you turn to watch the medball fly.

MEDBALL PUSH FROM KNEES

On paper, this looks so easy. After all, how hard can it be to push a 4–8-pound medball into the air? The answer: plenty hard. You'll need to produce a controlled, explosive, upper-body effort to launch the medball. With practice, you'll strengthen and stabilize your entire upper body and core. Also, final launch position requires a full triple extension of your hip, knees, and ankles that isn't far removed from first-steps acceleration.

221

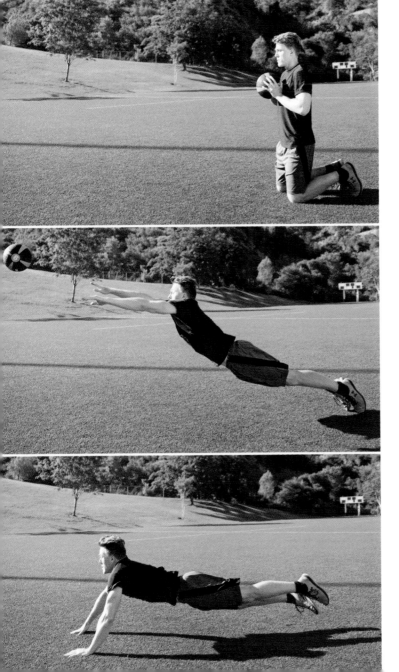

WORKOUT 3–5 reps

▸ Begin in a kneeling position. Hold the medball at chest height, with your elbows resting against your sides. Maintain a straight back, with your eyes forward.

▸ Thrust the medball out from your chest, simultaneously bringing your hips forward—your knees will rise off the ground.

▸ Expect momentum to carry you forward, so that you fall on the ground.

PUSH-UPS

The Push-Up is a simple, effective exercise for developing triceps, chest, and shoulder strength, not to mention providing a great core workout. While not explosive like Medball Push from Knees or Plyo Push-Ups, this exercise helps you develop the basic muscle strength and neural pathways that will make those explosive exercises possible.

222

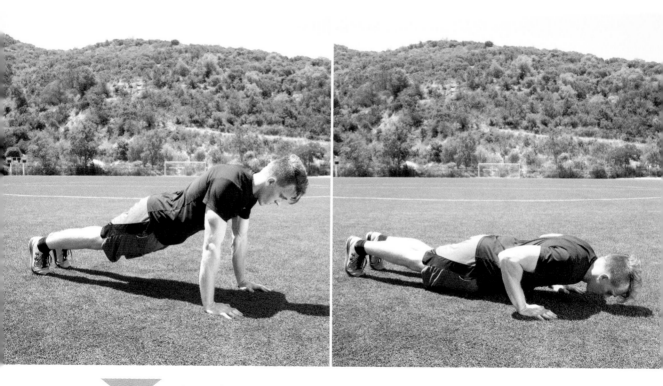

WORKOUT   **1–2 sets of 5–25 reps**

▸ Start at the top of the push-up position: arms extended beneath your shoulders, spine and legs straight, weight distributed on your toes and hands, eyes looking at the ground.

▸ Bend your elbows to lower yourself toward the ground (don't touch—no resting!).

▸ Push against the ground to rise back to your starting position.

PUSH-UPS WITH MEDBALL

This variation on the traditional Push-Up creates a challenge for your core stabilization ability. By preventing full extension of one arm (the medball-side arm), you'll keep the same-side triceps, chest, and shoulder muscles activated continuously—a reason for limiting the number of repetitions you perform.

223

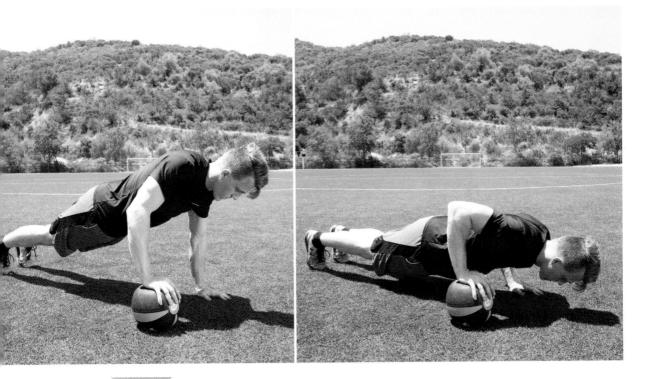

WORKOUT **2 sets of 5–15 reps, switching medball hand after first set**

▶ Begin at the top of a push-up position, with right arm fully extended beneath your shoulder and left hand on medball. Your left elbow should be bent enough to create a level plane across your shoulders, and your feet a little wider apart than they'd be for a regular push-up.

▶ Lower your chest until it's 1–2 inches off the ground.

▶ Return to start position, retaining a level plane across your shoulders at all times.

▶ Finish reps for the left hand, then switch to your right hand for the second set.

COACH'S 2 CENTS

If you become proficient at both this exercise and Plyo Push-Ups, combine them by flicking the ball toward your opposite hand each time you explode upward, then land with one hand on the ground, one on the ball; next, do the medball push-up, then explode and flick again.

PLYO PUSH-UPS

This variation on a traditional Push-Up adds a plyometric twist. You'll use an explosive push from your triceps, chest, and shoulders to propel your torso off the ground. As you land, you'll use eccentric contractions of those same muscles to store elastic energy and create a strength-shortening cycle to fuel your next upward explosion.

224

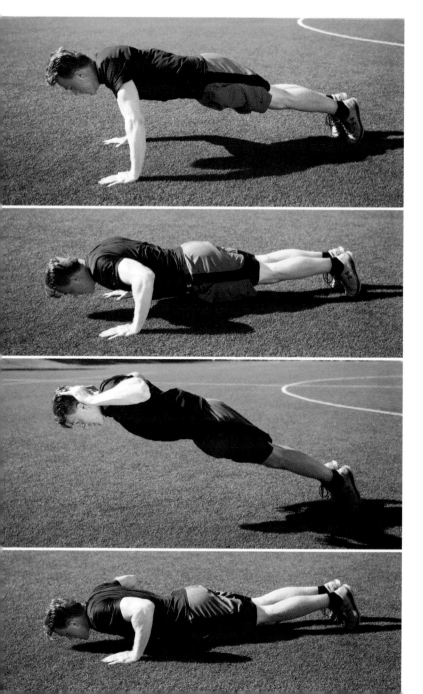

WORKOUT **1–2 sets of 5–10 reps**

▶ Begin at the top of a traditional push-up position—arms extended beneath your shoulders, spine straight, on your toes.

▶ Lower your chest toward the ground.

▶ Explode upward, pushing hard enough to create space between your hands and the ground.

▶ Land on your hands, partially arresting your momentum. As you're about to touch the ground again, explode upward once more.

COACH'S 2 CENTS

Don't come to a complete stop as you lower yourself to the ground, and don't lower too slowly—you need the movement to occur quickly to store elastic energy and then use it. Also, this exercise can be tough on the wrists, so limit reps and sessions accordingly.

RUSSIAN OBLIQUE TWIST

With the Russian Oblique Twist, you'll strengthen the muscles that border your six-pack and help control torso rotation and side bends. Strengthening your obliques will improve your stability, reduce pressure on your lower back, and improve your posture.

225

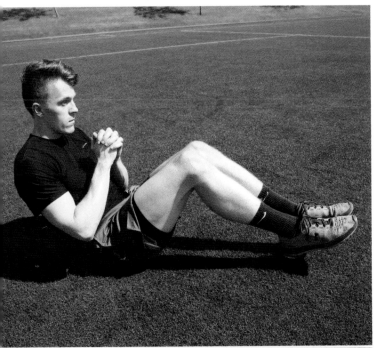

WORKOUT   **1–2 sets of 10–15 reps each side**

▸ Begin in a sitting position. Raise your heels off the ground and clasp your hands in front of your chest, balancing on your butt.

▸ Keep your hips and legs stable as you twist your upper body to the right and touch your clasped hands to the ground (or as close as you can get).

▸ Repeat the previous steps to the left.

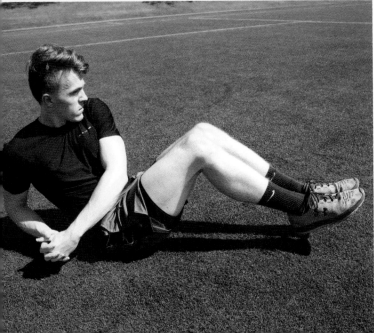

COACH'S 2 CENTS

Keep your eyes forward and your neck and shoulders loose throughout the exercise.

MONSTER WALK

Ever seen the old Frankenstein movie starring Boris Karloff? If so, you'll know where this gets its name. Physical therapists love this exercise because it strengthens the entire kinetic chain (the interconnected chain of connective tissue, muscles, and nerves that are affected by the movement of a member of the chain). You'll work your glutes and hip abductors specifically, with benefits for stability up and down your legs.

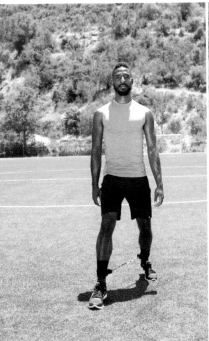 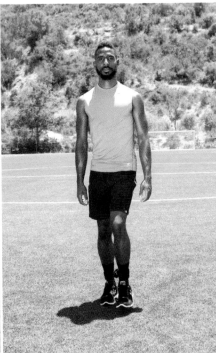 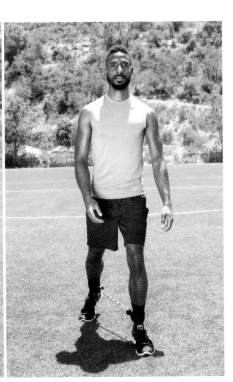

WORKOUT   **1-2 sets of 10-20 steps (total for both legs)**

▶ Secure a resistance band or tubing above your knees or around your ankles. Stand with feet hip-width apart, knees slightly bent, arms hanging loose at your sides.

▶ Step forward and out with your right leg—at about a 45° angle from your start position. Keep the bend in your knees and arms at your sides as you move.

▶ Step forward and to the opposite side (45°) with your left leg.

▶ Step again with your right leg, bringing that leg back to the center position as you move forward before angling to the side (45°) again.

▶ Continue stepping for the remainder of the exercise.

COACH'S 2 CENTS

As you move your leg inward before angling out 45°, ensure your knees don't buckle inward—the whole leg should move as a single, stable unit. For best muscle activation, the resistance band should be looped around your ankles. Looping above or below your knees provides less activation. Pick the location that works best for you.

SIDE STEPS WITH RESISTANCE BAND

After doing basic hip abductor strengthening with Side Leg Lifts or Side Steps (Quick), you're ready to up the intensity by using a resistance band.

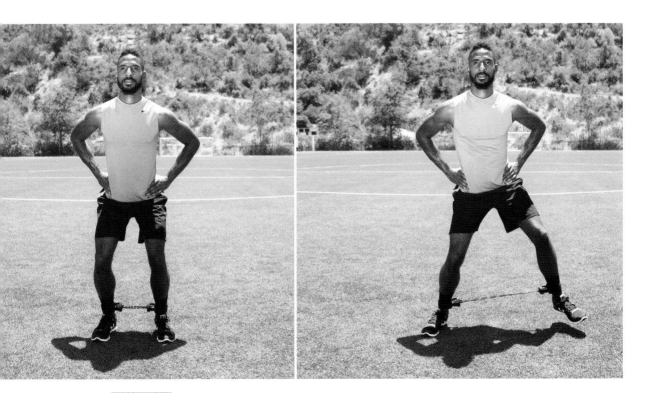

▼ **WORKOUT** **1–2 sets of 10–20 side steps
(half in one direction, half in reverse)**

▶ Secure a resistance band (or resistance tubing) above your knees or around your ankles. Stand with feet hip-width apart, knees slightly bent, hands on your hips.

▶ Step to the right until you feel significant resistance from the band.

▶ Slide your left foot over to recreate your original stance.

▶ Continue for half your reps, then switch directions for the second half.

COACH'S 2 CENTS

For best muscle activation, the resistance band should be looped around your ankles. No yanking the resistance band or letting it yank you—practice a smooth controlled motion both when side-stepping and recreating the original stance.

STEP-UPS

Step-Ups target concentric contractions of your glutes and hamstrings. By starting this exercise with your knee and hip at 90 degrees, you mimic the "push" dynamics of your hip and knee joints during first-steps acceleration—this is a good way to develop special strength for acceleration.

228

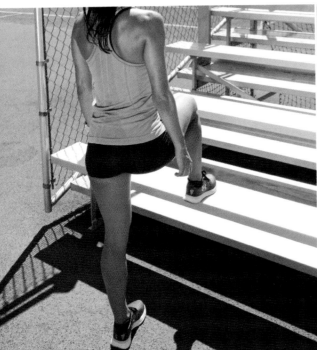
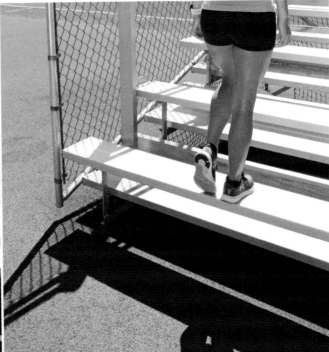

WORKOUT   **2–3 sets of 5–10 reps for each leg**

▸ Stand in front of a platform (e.g., a bench or step). Place your right foot on the platform, with your left foot flat on the ground.

▸ With your arms at your sides, push with your right leg (quadriceps and hip extensors) to extend your hip and knee and rise onto the platform.

▸ Rest the ball of your left foot on the platform. After a short pause, reverse direction to return to your starting position.

▸ Do all your repetitions with your right leg, then switch legs.

COACH'S 2 CENTS

Never start with your knee or hip angles greater than 90°—it places too great a strain on the muscles that control movement at those joints (and on the joints themselves).

STEP-DOWNS

Step-Downs work your quadriceps muscles eccentrically, strengthening them in preparation for the load they'll encounter when your foot touches down during each stride.

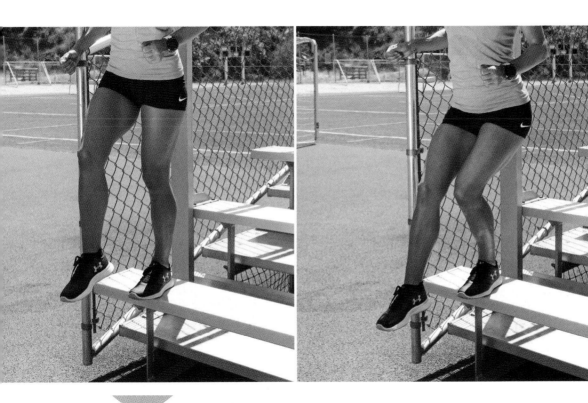

WORKOUT **1–2 sets of 5–10 reps each**

▸ Balance on one foot at the edge of a platform (e.g., a step or plyo box), holding onto a nearby object for balance if needed. Suspend the opposite leg, knee bent, in front of the platform.

▸ Lower your hips by bending your support knee to approximately 45°.

▸ Rise back to your starting position. Repeat.

▸ Switch legs once you've finished your total reps for that set.

HEEL DIPS

Heel Dips were discovered by Swedish orthopedist Håkan Alfredson. He tried to rupture his own chronically injured Achilles tendons with hundreds of heel dips per day. He did this because he wanted to force his reluctant clinic supervisor to perform surgery on his Achilles. Instead, Alfredson cured himself. Sprinting requires massive storage of elastic energy in your Achilles tendons, and stiffer tendons are key to achieving that goal. Heel Dips will give you stiffer tendons and protect you from Achilles injuries.

230

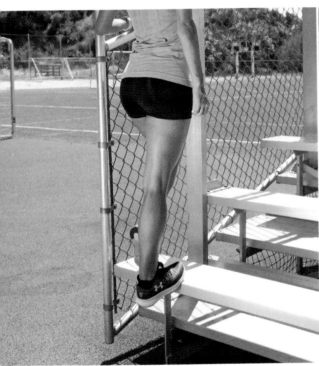 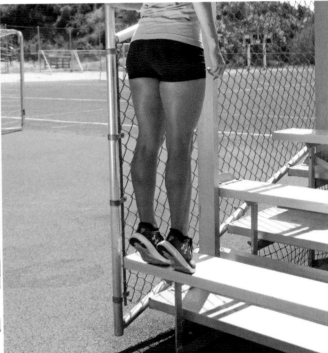

WORKOUT 2–3 sets of 5–20 reps

▶ Balance on the balls of your feet on a platform or step. Your heels should extend over the edge of the platform. Use a rail or other support for balance.

▶ Shift all your weight to your right foot and slowly lower your right heel through your full range of motion.

▶ Use both feet to quickly rise back to the balls of your feet.

▶ Do all reps on one foot, and then switch to the other.

COACH'S 2 CENTS

This isn't about working your calves—it's about the effect that lowering your heel has on your Achilles tendon. Don't take too long to lower your heel; if you're taking longer than one second, pick up the pace. If the exercise becomes easy, wear a weight vest or hold a dumbbell in the same-side hand as the exercising heel while performing your dips. Also, if a platform or step isn't available, or if pain or stiffness prevents dropping your heel below ground level, it's okay to perform these on the ground, lowering your heel to the ground before rising back on your toes.

10

SPEEDRUNNER SCHEDULES

Core Schedule: Four weeks of training to develop acceleration, maximum velocity, strength, agility, balance, and proprioception

Speed-Only Schedule: Four weeks of training for athletes focused on developing acceleration and maximum velocity; suggested for those who already include strength and agility training in their fitness or sports programs

Distance Runner Once-Per-Week Schedule: For distance runners (and other endurance athletes) who want to improve their leg speed but already have full training schedules

Solo Sessions: Aimed at athletes who've completed the Core schedule and are seeking extra training, these sessions target specific aspects of your speed, strength, and agility training, including:

- Acceleration
- Maximum velocity
- Whole-body strength
- Core muscles and hips
- Injury prevention

Each schedule lists the day's exercises and drills in order and the suggested recovery between reps, drills, and exercises. Appendix A contains an important table for metrics testing. It consists of four basic tests, listed in order, that allow you to organize your pre- and post-SpeedRunner testing. Test yourself before you start a SpeedRunner schedule and again after to see how you've improved.

Appendix B lists all the prop, no-prop, and prop swap options. Prop exercises have "No-Props" alternatives (if available), with additional information on "prop swaps." Prop swaps are everyday items you can use to replace a prop, making it possible to perform the "Props" version of the exercise even if you don't have access to the designated prop.

GUIDELINES FOR USING THE SPEEDRUNNER SCHEDULES

THE SPEEDRUNNER SCHEDULES work best if you adhere to the specific guidelines for each schedule. As you read the guidelines, which precede each schedule, remember that the best workouts are those that stimulate the most useful and comprehensive adaptations. "Feeling the burn" won't make you a better athlete. Getting faster, stronger, and quicker will make you a better athlete. So resist the urge to train harder than necessary. If the sessions feel too easy, you can always create more challenging sessions after your Core training. First, though, try it the SpeedRunner way.

CORE SCHEDULE

✔ Four weeks

✔ Three sessions per week
  ▸ **1st session:** Acceleration & Strength
  ▸ **2nd session:** Agility & Strength
  ▸ **3rd session:** Maximum Velocity

✔ One recovery day between sessions

✔ Two recovery days between the third session of one week and the first session of the next week (if you add a speed endurance day, it should come the day after a Core session and must be followed by a day off)

✔ Strength Circuit exercises refer to groups of exercises that follow the circuit-training format: one circuit equals the completion of one set of all prescribed exercises, in order (repeat the circuit the number of times indicated)

✔ Any concurrent training (e.g., team sports practice) must be low-intensity

A sample week of the Core schedule might look like this:

MON.	TUES.	WED.	THURS.	FRI.	SAT.	SUN.
Session 1 Acceleration & Strength	Recovery	**Session 2** Agility & Strength	Recovery	**Session 3** Maximum Velocity	Speed Endurance Day	Recovery

WEEK 1

234

	PROPS	NO PROPS
WARM-UP	**WARM-UP**	
	Buildups 4-2-2 (p. 123)	Buildups 4-2-2 (p. 123)

Strength Circuit 1 | Technique Drills

	Strength Circuit 1	
	▸ **2 CIRCUITS**	▸ **2 CIRCUITS**
	Air Squats (p. 194), *5–10 reps*	Air Squats (p. 194), *5–10 reps*
	Push-Ups (p. 222), *5–10 reps*	Push-Ups (p. 222), *5–10 reps*
	Russian Oblique Twist (p. 225), *10 reps each side*	Russian Oblique Twist (p. 225), *10 reps each side*
	30 sec. rest between exercises, 1 min. rest between circuits	**30 sec. rest between exercises, 1 min. rest between circuits**

STRIDES	**STRIDES**	
	Strides (90%) (p. 182), *2 reps*	Strides (90%) (p. 182), *2 reps*

Acceleration | Agility | Maximum Velocity

	Acceleration Exercises	
	Push-Up & Sprint (p. 132), *2 reps*	Push-Up & Sprint (p. 132), *2 reps*
	Standing Broad Jump (p. 187), *2 reps*	Standing Broad Jump (p. 187), *2 reps*
	Standing Starts (forward sprints only) (p. 133), *2 sets*	Standing Starts (forward sprints only) (p. 133), *2 sets*
	1–2 min. rest after each rep, 3 min. rest before Strength Circuit 2	**1–2 min. rest after each rep, 3 min. rest before Strength Circuit 2**

Strength Circuit 2

	Strength Circuit 2	
	▸ **2 CIRCUITS**	▸ **2 CIRCUITS**
	Step-Downs (p. 229), *5 reps each side*	Step-Downs (p. 229), *5 reps each side*
	Single-Leg Deadlift (p. 208), *5 reps each side*	Single-Leg Deadlift (p. 208), *5 reps each side*
	Heel Dips (p. 230), *10 reps each side*	Heel Dips (p. 230), *10 reps each side*
	30 sec. rest between exercises, 1 min. rest between circuits	**30 sec. rest between exercises, 1 min. rest between circuits**

FINAL EXERCISE	**FINAL EXERCISE**	
	Bear Crawl (p. 196), *2 × 20 yd.*	Bear Crawl (p. 196), *2 × 20 yd.*
	3 min. rest between reps	**3 min. rest between reps**

Add 1 day of recovery between sessions and 2 days of recovery between the 3rd session of one week and the 1st session of the next week. The elective Speed Endurance day (see pages 97–102) should come after a Core session and should be followed by a day off.

SESSION 2 **AGILITY & STRENGTH**		SESSION 3 **MAXIMUM VELOCITY**	
PROPS	**NO PROPS**	**PROPS**	**NO PROPS**
WARM-UP		**WARM-UP**	
Buildups 4-2-2 (p. 123)	Buildups 4-2-2 (p. 123)	Jogging (p. 122), *10–15 min.*	Jogging (p. 122), *10–15 min.*
Strength Circuit 1		**Technique Drills**	
▸ **2 CIRCUITS**	▸ **2 CIRCUITS**	Skipping (p. 164)	Skipping (p. 164)
Push-Ups with Medball (p. 223), *5 reps each side*	Push-Ups with Medball (use prop swap) (p. 223), *5 reps each side*	High Skipping (p. 165)	High Skipping (p. 165)
Plank (p. 204), *30 sec.*	Plank (p. 204), *30 sec.*	Flat-Footed Marching (p. 166)	Flat-Footed Marching (p. 166)
Side Steps (Quick) (p. 149), *15 yd. each direction*	Side Steps (Quick) (p. 149), *15 yd. each direction*	High Knees (p. 167)	High Knees (p. 167)
30 sec. rest between exercises, 1 min. rest between circuits	30 sec. rest between exercises, 1 min. rest between circuits	Quick Feet (p. 168)	Quick Feet (p. 168)
		Butt Kicks (p. 170)	Butt Kicks (p. 170)
STRIDES		After each drill, jog back to start, stride at 90% effort same distance as drill, walk back to start	After each drill, jog back to start, stride at 90% effort same distance as drill, walk back to start
Strides (90%) (p. 182), *2 reps*	Strides (90%) (p. 182), *2 reps*		
Agility Exercises		**Maximum Velocity Exercises**	
Agility Ladder 3 Quick Steps (p. 144), *2 reps*	3-Step, 1-Step (p. 148), *2 reps*	Ankle Poppers (p. 178), *15 sec. each foot, 2 reps*	Ankle Poppers (p. 178), *15 sec., 2 reps*
Agility Ladder 2-Legged Hops (p. 142), *2 reps*	Agility Ladder 2-Legged Hops (use prop swap) (p. 142), *10 hops, 2 sets*	Weighted Ankle Poppers (p. 179), *30 sec. each foot, 2 reps*	Weighted Ankle Poppers (use prop swap) (p. 179), *30 sec. each foot, 2 reps*
Backward Running (p. 150), *20 yd., 2 reps*	Backward Running (p. 150), *20 yd., 2 reps*	Triple Hop on 1 Leg (p. 172), *2 reps each side*	Triple Hop on 1 Leg (p. 172), *2 reps each side*
1–2 min. rest after each rep, 3 min. rest before Strength Circuit 2	1–2 min. rest after each rep, 3 min. rest before Strength Circuit 2	2–3 min. rest after each rep	2–3 min. rest after each rep
Strength Circuit 2			
▸ **2 CIRCUITS**	▸ **2 CIRCUITS**		
Nordic Curls (p. 202), *5 reps* (or Single-Leg Deadlifts (p. 208), *5 reps each side*)	Nordic Curls (p. 202), *5 reps* (or Single-Leg Deadlifts (p. 208), *5 reps each side*)		
Leg Lifts (p. 200), *20 reps*	Leg Lifts (p. 200), *20 reps*		
Hip Thrusts (with bench) (p. 214), *3–5 reps*	Hip Thrusts (ground level) (p. 215), *3–5 reps*		
30 sec. rest between exercises, 1 min. rest between circuits	30 sec. rest between exercises, 1 min. rest between circuits		
FINAL EXERCISE		**FINAL EXERCISE**	
20-Yard Square (p. 154), *2 reps*	20-Yard Square (p. 154), *2 reps*	Strides (95%) (p. 182), *65–75 yd., 2 reps*	Strides (95%) (p. 182), *65–75 yd., 2 reps*
3 min. rest between reps	3 min. rest between reps		

236

WEEK 2

SESSION 1
ACCELERATION & STRENGTH

PROPS	NO PROPS

WARM-UP

WARM-UP

Buildups 4-2-2 (p. 123)	Buildups 4-2-2 (p. 123)

Strength Circuit 1 | Technique Drills

Strength Circuit 1

▶ **2 CIRCUITS**	▶ **2 CIRCUITS**
Jump Squats (p. 174), *5–10 reps*	Jump Squats (p. 174), *5–10 reps*
Battle Ropes (p. 218), *30 sec.*	Push-Ups (p. 222), *10 reps*
Windshield Wipers (p. 212), *5–10 reps each side*	Windshield Wipers (p. 212), *5–10 reps each side*
30 sec. rest between exercises, 1 min. rest between circuits	**30 sec. rest between exercises, 1 min. rest between circuits**

STRIDES

STRIDES

Strides (90%) (p. 182), *2 reps*	Strides (90%) (p. 182), *2 reps*

Acceleration | Agility | Maximum Velocity

Acceleration Exercises

Medball Push & Sprint (p. 131), *2 reps*	Jump & Sprint (p. 128), *2 reps*
Standing 5-Jump (p. 134), *2 sets of 5 jumps*	Standing 5-Jump (p. 134), *2 sets of 5 jumps*
Weight Sled Marching (p. 136), *15 yd., 2 reps*	Stadium Steps Marching (p. 130), *15 sec., 2 reps*
1–2 min. rest after each rep, 3 min. rest before Strength Circuit 2	**1–2 min. rest after each rep, 3 min. rest before Strength Circuit 2**

Strength Circuit 2

Strength Circuit 2

▶ **2 CIRCUITS**	▶ **2 CIRCUITS**
Lunge Clock (p. 216), *1 revolution (switch direction for second circuit)*	Lunge Clock (p. 216), *1 revolution (switch direction for second circuit)*
Single-Leg Deadlift (p. 208), *8–10 reps each side*	Single-Leg Deadlift (p. 208), *8–10 reps each side*
Heel Dips (p. 230), *15 reps each side*	Heel Dips (p. 230), *15 reps each side*
30 sec. rest between exercises, 1 min. rest between circuits	**30 sec. rest between exercises, 1 min. rest between circuits**

FINAL EXERCISE

FINAL EXERCISE

Resisted Run (p. 129), *2 × 10 sec.* **2 min. rest between reps**	Mountain Climbers (p. 203), *2 × 20 sec.* **2 min. rest between reps**

Add 1 day of recovery between sessions and 2 days of recovery between the 3rd session of one week and the 1st session of the next week. The elective Speed Endurance day (see pages 97–102) should come after a Core session and should be followed by a day off.

SESSION 2 AGILITY & STRENGTH		SESSION 3 MAXIMUM VELOCITY	
PROPS	**NO PROPS**	**PROPS**	**NO PROPS**
WARM-UP		**WARM-UP**	
Buildups 4-2-2 (p. 123)	Buildups 4-2-2 (p. 123)	Jogging (p. 122), *10–15 min.*	Jogging (p. 122), *10–15 min.*
Strength Circuit 1		**Technique Drills**	
▸ **2 CIRCUITS** Push-Ups with Medball (p. 223), *5–10 reps each side* Plank (p. 204), *30 sec.* Side Steps (Quick) (p. 149), *15 yd. each direction* 30 sec. rest between exercises, 1 min. rest between circuits	▸ **2 CIRCUITS** Push-Ups with Medball (use prop swap) (p. 223), *5–10 reps each side* Plank (p. 204), *30 sec.* Side Steps (Quick) (p. 149), *15 yd. each direction* 30 sec. rest between exercises, 1 min. rest between circuits	Skipping (p. 164) High Skipping (p. 165) Flat-Footed Marching (p. 166) Bounding (p. 127) High Knees (p. 167) Quick Feet (p. 168) Butt Kicks (p. 170) After each drill, jog back to start, stride at 90% effort same distance as drill, walk back to start	Skipping (p. 164) High Skipping (p. 165) Flat-Footed Marching (p. 166) Bounding (p. 127) High Knees (p. 167) Quick Feet (p. 168) Butt Kicks (p. 170) After each drill, jog back to start, stride at 90% effort same distance as drill, walk back to start
STRIDES			
Strides (90%) (p. 182), *2 reps*	Strides (90%) (p. 182), *2 reps*		
Agility Exercises		**Maximum Velocity Exercises**	
Agility Ladder Step In 'n' Out (p. 146), *1 rep each direction* Agility Ladder 1-Legged Hops (p. 140), *1 rep each leg* Standing Starts (p. 133), *1 set of all 6 sprints* 1–2 min. rest after each rep, 3 min. rest before Strength Circuit 2	Step Back 'n' Forth Drill (p. 147), *1 rep each direction* Agility Ladder 1-Legged Hops (use prop swap) (p. 141), *10 hops each leg* Standing Starts (p. 133), *1 set of all 6 sprints* 1–2 min. rest after each rep, 3 min. rest before Strength Circuit 2	Ankle Poppers (p. 178), *15 sec. each foot, 2 reps* Weighted Ankle Poppers (p. 179), *30 sec. each foot, 2 reps* Depth Jumps (p. 173), *3 reps* 2–3 min. rest after each rep	Ankle Poppers (p. 178), *15 sec. each foot, 2 reps* Weighted Ankle Poppers (use prop swap) (p. 179), *30 sec. each foot, 2 reps* Double-Leg Hops (p. 180), *3 reps* 2–3 min. rest after each rep
Strength Circuit 2			
▸ **2 CIRCUITS** Nordic Curls (p. 202), *8 reps* (or Single-Leg Deadlifts (p. 208), *8 reps each side*) V-Ups with Medball (p. 211), *5–10 reps* Hip Thrusts (with bench) (p. 214), *5–10 reps* 30 sec. rest between exercises, 1 min. rest between circuits	▸ **2 CIRCUITS** Nordic Curls (p. 202), *8 reps* (or Single-Leg Deadlifts (p. 208), *8 reps each side*) V-Ups (p. 211), *5–10 reps* Hip Thrusts (ground level) (p. 215), *5–10 reps* 30 sec. rest between exercises, 1 min. rest between circuits		
FINAL EXERCISE		**FINAL EXERCISE**	
Figure 8 Drill (p. 156), *2 reps* 3 min. rest between reps	Figure 8 Drill (p. 156), *2 reps* 3 min. rest between reps	Hill Sprints and Stadium Steps (p. 130), *2 reps* 1 min. rest between reps	Hill Sprints and Stadium Steps (p. 130), *2 reps* 1 min. rest between reps

WEEK 3

SESSION 1
ACCELERATION & STRENGTH

PROPS	NO PROPS
WARM-UP	
WARM-UP	
Buildups 4-2-2 (p. 123)	Buildups 4-2-2 (p. 123)

WARM-UP

Strength Circuit 1 | Technique Drills

Strength Circuit 1

PROPS	NO PROPS
▸ **2 CIRCUITS**	▸ **2 CIRCUITS**
Jump Squats with Weight (p. 175), *5–10 reps*	Jump Squats (p. 174), *5–10 reps*
Battle Ropes (p. 218), *30 sec.*	Plank Rotations (p. 205), *5–10 reps each side*
Russian Oblique Twist (p. 225), *10 reps each side*	Russian Oblique Twist (p. 225), *10 reps each side*
30 sec. rest between exercises, 1 min. rest between circuits	**30 sec. rest between exercises, 1 min. rest between circuits**

STRIDES

STRIDES

PROPS	NO PROPS
Strides (90%) (p. 182), *2 reps*	Strides (90%) (p. 182), *2 reps*

Acceleration | Agility | Maximum Velocity

Acceleration Exercises

PROPS	NO PROPS
Weight Sled Push (p. 135), *10 yd., 2 reps*	3-Bounce & Run (p. 124), *2 reps*
3-Bounce & Run (p. 124), *2 reps*	Hill Sprints and Stadium Steps (p. 130), *2 reps*
Weight Sled Run (p. 138), *20 yds., 2 reps*	Downhill Sprints or 30-yd. sprints (95%) if no hill (p. 130), *2 reps*
1–2 min. rest after each rep, 3 min. rest before Strength Circuit 2	**1–2 min. rest after each rep, 3 min. rest before Strength Circuit 2**

Strength Circuit 2

Strength Circuit 2

PROPS	NO PROPS
▸ **2 CIRCUITS**	▸ **2 CIRCUITS**
Step-Downs (p. 229), *8–10 reps each side*	Step-Downs (p. 229), *8–10 reps each side*
Heel Dips (p. 230), *15–20 reps each side*	Heel Dips (p. 230), *15–20 reps each side*
Single-Leg Squats (p. 207), *3–5 reps each side*	Single-Leg Squats (p. 207), *3–5 reps each side*
30 sec. rest between exercises, 1 min. rest between circuits	**30 sec. rest between exercises, 1 min. rest between circuits**

FINAL EXERCISE

FINAL EXERCISE

PROPS	NO PROPS
Overhead Medball Throw (p. 220), *3 reps*	Crab Walk (p. 197), *2 × 10 yd.*
1 min. rest between reps	**3 min. rest between reps**

Add 1 day of recovery between sessions and 2 days of recovery between the 3rd session of one week and the 1st session of the next week. The elective Speed Endurance day (see pages 97–102) should come after a Core session and should be followed by a day off.

SESSION 2 **AGILITY & STRENGTH**		SESSION 3 **MAXIMUM VELOCITY**	
PROPS	**NO PROPS**	**PROPS**	**NO PROPS**
WARM-UP		**WARM-UP**	
Buildups 4-2-2 (p. 123)	Buildups 4-2-2 (p. 123)	Jogging (p. 122), *10–15 min.*	Jogging (p. 122), *10–15 min.*
Strength Circuit 1		**Technique Drills**	
▸ **2 CIRCUITS**	▸ **2 CIRCUITS**	Skipping (p. 164)	Skipping (p. 164)
Medball Push from Knees (p. 221), *1 rep per circuit (add 1 more rep at end of circuits]*	Plyo Push-Ups (p. 224), *5 reps*	High Skipping (p. 165)	High Skipping (p. 165)
		Flat-Footed Marching (p. 166)	Flat-Footed Marching (p. 166)
Bird Dogs (p. 198), *5–10 reps each side*	Bird Dogs (p. 198), *5–10 reps each side*	Bounding (p. 127)	Bounding (p. 127)
		High Knees (p. 167)	High Knees (p. 167)
Weight Sled Crossover (p. 160), *10 yd., reverse direction for 2nd circuit*	Stadium Crossover Steps (p. 161), *5–10 steps, reverse front/back leg for 2nd rep*	Quick Feet (p. 168)	Quick Feet (p. 168)
		Quick Hops (p. 169)	Quick Hops (p. 169)
		Butt Kicks (p. 170)	Butt Kicks (p. 170)
30 sec. rest between exercises, 1 min. rest between circuits	30 sec. rest between exercises, 1 min. rest between circuits	After each drill, jog back to start, stride at 90% effort same distance as drill, walk back to start	After each drill, jog back to start, stride at 90% effort same distance as drill, walk back to start
STRIDES			
Strides (90%) (p. 182), *2 reps*	Strides (90%) (p. 182), *2 reps*		
Agility Exercises		**Maximum Velocity Exercises**	
Agility Ladder 3 Quick Steps (p. 144), *2 reps*	3-Step, 1-Step (p. 148), *2 reps*	Ankle Poppers (p. 178), *15 sec. each foot, 2 reps*	Ankle Poppers (p. 178), *15 sec. each foot, 2 reps*
Agility Ladder Ickey Shuffle (p. 145), *2 reps*	Agility Ladder Ickey Shuffle (use prop swap) (p. 145), *2 reps*	Walking Lunges (p. 176), *5 lunges each side, 2 reps*	Walking Lunges (p. 176), *5 lunges each side, 2 reps*
Backward Running (p. 150), *20 yd., 2 reps*	Backward Running (p. 150), *20 yd., 2 reps*	Triple Hop on 1 Leg (p. 172), *2 reps each leg*	Triple Hop on 1 Leg (p. 172), *2 reps each leg*
1–2 min. rest after each rep, 3 min. rest before Strength Circuit 2	1–2 min. rest after each rep, 3 min. rest before Strength Circuit 2	2–3 min. rest after each rep	2–3 min. rest after each rep
Strength Circuit 2			
▸ **2 CIRCUITS**	▸ **2 CIRCUITS**		
Nordic Curls (p. 202), *10 reps [or Single-Leg Deadlifts (p. 208), 10 reps each side]*	Nordic Curls (p. 202), *10 reps [or Single-Leg Deadlifts (p. 208), 10 reps each side]*		
Leg Lifts (p. 200), *20 reps*	Leg Lifts (p. 200), *20 reps*		
Hip Thrusts (with bench) (p. 214), *5–10 reps*	Hip Thrusts (ground level) (p. 215), *5–10 reps*		
30 sec. rest between exercises, 1 min. rest between circuits	30 sec. rest between exercises, 1 min. rest between circuits		
FINAL EXERCISE		**FINAL EXERCISE**	
W-Pattern Cone Drill (p. 158), *1 rep each direction*	W-Pattern Cone Drill (p. 158), *1 rep each direction*	Strides (95%) (p. 182), *65–75 yd., 2 reps*	Strides (95%) (p. 182), *65–75 yd., 2 reps*
3 min. rest between reps	3 min. rest between reps		

WEEK 4

SESSION 1
ACCELERATION & STRENGTH

	PROPS	NO PROPS
WARM-UP	**WARM-UP**	
	Buildups 4-2-2 (p. 123)	Buildups 4-2-2 (p. 123)

Strength Circuit 1 | Technique Drills

Strength Circuit 1

PROPS	NO PROPS
▸ **2 CIRCUITS**	▸ **2 CIRCUITS**
Walking Lunges with Weight (p. 177), *5 lunges each side*	Walking Lunges (p. 176), *5 lunges each side*
Battle Ropes (p. 218), *30 sec.*	Plank Rotations (p. 205), *5–10 reps each side*
Kneeling Partner Medball Twist (p. 213), *30 sec.* [or Windshield Wipers (p. 212), *10 reps each side*]	Kneeling Partner Medball Twist (p. 213), *30 sec.* [or Windshield Wipers (p. 212), *10 reps each side*]
30 sec. rest between exercises, 1 min. rest between circuits	**30 sec. rest between exercises, 1 min. rest between circuits**

STRIDES

STRIDES

PROPS	NO PROPS
Strides (90%) (p. 182), *2 reps*	Strides (90%) (p. 182), *2 reps*

Acceleration | Agility | Maximum Velocity

Acceleration Exercises

PROPS	NO PROPS
Weight Sled Push (p. 135), *10–20 yd., 2 reps*	3-Point Stance & Sprint (p. 126), *2 reps*
3-Point Stance & Sprint (p. 126), *2 reps*	Hill Sprints and Stadium Steps (p. 130), *2 reps*
Weight Sled Run (p. 138), *20 yd., 2 reps*	Downhill Sprints or 30-yd. sprints (95%) if no hill (p. 130), *2 reps*
1–2 min. rest after each rep, 3 min. rest before Strength Circuit 2	**1–2 min. rest after each rep, 3 min. rest before Strength Circuit 2**

Strength Circuit 2

Strength Circuit 2

PROPS	NO PROPS
▸ **2 CIRCUITS**	▸ **2 CIRCUITS**
Lunge Clock (p. 216), *1 revolution (switch direction for second circuit)*	Lunge Clock (p. 216), *1 revolution (switch direction for second circuit)*
Heel Dips (p. 230), *15–20 reps each side*	Heel Dips (p. 230), *15–20 reps each side*
Single-Leg Squats (p. 207), *3–5 reps each side*	Single-Leg Squats (p. 207), *3–5 reps each side*
30 sec. rest between exercises, 1 min. rest between circuits	**30 sec. rest between exercises, 1 min. rest between circuits**

FINAL EXERCISE

FINAL EXERCISE

PROPS	NO PROPS
Tug Rope with Weight Sled or Weights (p. 217), *3 reps*	Pull-Ups (p. 217), *2 sets of maximum pull-up reps*
3 min. rest between reps	**3 min. rest between reps**

Add 1 day of recovery between sessions and 2 days of recovery between the 3rd session of one week and the 1st session of the next week. The elective Speed Endurance day (see pages 97–102) should come after a Core session and should be followed by a day off.

SESSION 2		SESSION 3	
AGILITY & STRENGTH		**MAXIMUM VELOCITY**	
PROPS	**NO PROPS**	**PROPS**	**NO PROPS**
WARM-UP		**WARM-UP**	
Buildups 4-2-2 [p. 123]	Buildups 4-2-2 [p. 123]	Jogging [p. 122], *10–15 min.*	Jogging [p. 122], *10–15 min.*
Strength Circuit 1		**Technique Drills**	
▸ **2 CIRCUITS** Medball Push from Knees [p. 221], *1 rep per circuit (add 1 more rep at end of circuits)* Superman/Superwoman Plank [p. 210], *5–10 reps each side* Weight Sled Crossover [p. 160], *10 yd., reverse direction for 2nd circuit* 30 sec. rest between exercises, 1 min. rest between circuits	▸ **2 CIRCUITS** Plyo Push-Ups [p. 224], *5–10 reps* Superman/Superwoman Plank [p. 210], *5–10 reps each side* Stadium Crossover Steps [p. 161], *5–10 steps, reverse front/back leg for 2nd rep* 30 sec. rest between exercises, 1 min. rest between circuits	Skipping [p. 164] High Skipping [p. 165] Flat-Footed Marching [p. 166] Bounding [p. 127] High Knees [p. 167] Quick Feet [p. 168] Quick Hops [p. 169] Butt Kicks [p. 170] After each drill, jog back to start, stride at 90% effort same distance as drill, walk back to start	Skipping [p. 164] High Skipping [p. 165] Flat-Footed Marching [p. 166] Bounding [p. 127] High Knees [p. 167] Quick Feet [p. 168] Quick Hops [p. 169] Butt Kicks [p. 170] After each drill, jog back to start, stride at 90% effort same distance as drill, walk back to start
STRIDES			
Strides [90%] [p. 182], *2 reps*	Strides [90%] [p. 182], *2 reps*		
Agility Exercises		**Maximum Velocity Exercises**	
Agility Ladder Step In 'n' Out [p. 146], *1 rep each direction* Agility Ladder Ickey Shuffle [p. 145], *2 reps* Standing Starts [p. 133], *1 set of all 6 sprints* 1–2 min. rest after each rep, 3 min. rest before Strength Circuit 2	Step Back 'n' Forth Drill [p. 147], *1 rep each direction* Agility Ladder Ickey Shuffle [use prop swap] [p. 145], *2 reps* Standing Starts [p. 133], *1 set of all 6 sprints* 1–2 min. rest after each rep, 3 min. rest before Strength Circuit 2	Weighted Ankle Poppers [p. 179], *30 sec. each foot, 2 reps* Triple Hop on 1 Leg [p. 172], *2 reps each side* Depth Jumps [p. 173], *3 reps* 2–3 min. rest after each rep	Weighted Ankle Poppers [use prop swap] [p. 179], *30 sec. each foot, 2 reps* Triple Hop on 1 Leg [p. 172], *2 reps each side* Double-Leg Hops [p. 180], *3 reps or* Single-Leg Hops *(if you're ready)* [p. 181], *1–2 reps each leg* 2–3 min. rest after each rep
Strength Circuit 2			
▸ **2 CIRCUITS** Nordic Curls [p. 202], *10 reps (or* Single-Leg Deadlifts [p. 208], *10 reps each side)* V-Ups with Medball [p. 211], *5–10 reps* Hip Thrusts [single leg] [p. 215], *5 reps each side* 30 sec. rest between exercises, 1 min. rest between circuits	▸ **2 CIRCUITS** Nordic Curls [p. 202], *10 reps (or* Single-Leg Deadlifts [p. 208], *10 reps each side)* V-Ups [p. 211], *5–10 reps* Hip Thrusts [single leg] [p. 215], *5 reps each side* 30 sec. rest between exercises, 1 min. rest between circuits		
FINAL EXERCISE		**FINAL EXERCISE**	
Mini-Suicides [p. 151], *2 reps* 3 min. rest between reps	Mini-Suicides [p. 151], *2 reps* 3 min. rest between reps	Hill Sprints and Stadium Steps [p. 130], *4 reps* 1 min. rest between reps	Hill Sprints and Stadium Steps [p. 130], *4 reps* 1 min. rest between reps

SPEED-ONLY SCHEDULE

✔ Four weeks

✔ Two sessions per week
  ▸ **1st session:** Acceleration & Strength
  ▸ **2nd session:** Maximum Velocity

✔ One to three recovery days between sessions

✔ If you add a speed endurance day, plan for at least one recovery day before your next SpeedRunner session (one day prior to speed endurance is recommended, too)

✔ Strength Circuit exercises refer to groups of exercises that follow the circuit-training format: one circuit equals the completion of one set of all prescribed exercises, in order (repeat the circuit the number of times indicated)

A sample week of the Speed-Only schedule might look like this:

MON.	TUES.	WED.	THURS.	FRI.	SAT.	SUN.
Session 1 Acceleration & Strength	Recovery	Recovery	**Session 2** Maximum Velocity	Recovery	Speed Endurance Day	Recovery

WEEK 1

SESSION 1 ACCELERATION & STRENGTH		SESSION 2 MAXIMUM VELOCITY	
PROPS	**NO PROPS**	**PROPS**	**NO PROPS**
WARM-UP		WARM-UP	
Buildups 4-2-2 (p. 123)	Buildups 4-2-2 (p. 123)	Jogging (p. 122), 10–15 min.	Jogging (p. 122), 10–15 min.
Strength Circuit 1		**Technique Drills**	
▸ **2 CIRCUITS** Air Squats (p. 194), 5–10 reps Plank (p. 204), 30 sec. Step-Downs (p. 229), 5 reps each side 30 sec. rest between exercises, 1 min. rest between circuits	▸ **2 CIRCUITS** Air Squats (p. 194), 5–10 reps Plank (p. 204), 30 sec. Step-Downs (p. 229), 5 reps each side 30 sec. rest between exercises, 1 min. rest between circuits	Skipping (p. 164) High Skipping (p. 165) Flat-Footed Marching (p. 166) High Knees (p. 167) Quick Feet (p. 168) Butt Kicks (p. 170) **After each drill, jog back to start, stride at 90% effort same distance as drill, walk back to start**	Skipping (p. 164) High Skipping (p. 165) Flat-Footed Marching (p. 166) High Knees (p. 167) Quick Feet (p. 168) Butt Kicks (p. 170) **After each drill, jog back to start, stride at 90% effort same distance as drill, walk back to start**
STRIDES			
Strides (90%) (p. 182), 2 reps	Strides (90%) (p. 182), 2 reps		
Acceleration Exercises		**Maximum Velocity Exercises**	
Push-Up & Sprint (p. 132), 2 reps Standing Broad Jump (p. 187), 2 reps Standing Starts (forward sprints only) (p. 133), 2 sets 1–2 min. rest after each rep, 3 min. rest before Strength Circuit 2	Push-Up & Sprint (p. 132), 2 reps Standing Broad Jump (p. 187), 2 reps Standing Starts (forward sprints only) (p. 133), 2 sets 1–2 min. rest after each rep, 3 min. rest before Strength Circuit 2	Walking Lunges (p. 176), 5 lunges each side, 2 reps Leg Lifts (p. 200), 2 sets of 20 reps Heel Dips (p. 230), 2 sets of 10 reps each side Triple Hop on 1 Leg (p. 172), 2 reps each leg, alternating 2–3 min. rest after each rep	Walking Lunges (p. 176), 5 lunges each side, 2 reps Leg Lifts (p. 200), 2 sets of 20 reps Heel Dips (p. 230), 2 sets of 10 reps each side Triple Hop on 1 Leg (p. 172), 2 reps each leg, alternating 2–3 min. rest after each rep
Strength Circuit 2			
▸ **2 CIRCUITS** Heel Dips (p. 230), 10 reps each side Leg Lifts (p. 200), 10–20 reps Nordic Curls (p. 202), 5 reps (or Single-Leg Deadlifts (p. 208), 5 reps each side) 30 sec. rest between exercises, 1 min. rest between circuits	▸ **2 CIRCUITS** Heel Dips (p. 230), 10 reps each side Leg Lifts (p. 200), 10–20 reps Nordic Curls (p. 202), 5 reps (or Single-Leg Deadlifts (p. 208), 5 reps each side) 30 sec. rest between exercises, 1 min. rest between circuits		
FINAL EXERCISE		FINAL EXERCISE	
Bear Crawl (p. 196), 2 × 20 yd. 3 min. rest between reps	Bear Crawl (p. 196), 2 × 20 yd. 3 min. rest between reps	Strides (95%) (p. 182), 65–75 yd., 2 reps	Strides (95%) (p. 182), 65–75 yd., 2 reps

Build in 1–3 days of recovery between SpeedRunner sessions. The elective Speed Endurance day (see pages 97–102) should be followed by a day off.

WEEK 2

SESSION 1 ACCELERATION & STRENGTH		SESSION 2 MAXIMUM VELOCITY	
PROPS	**NO PROPS**	**PROPS**	**NO PROPS**
WARM-UP		**WARM-UP**	
Buildups 4-2-2 (p. 123)	Buildups 4-2-2 (p. 123)	Jogging (p. 122), 10–15 min.	Jogging (p. 122), 10–15 min.
Strength Circuit 1		**Technique Drills**	
▸ **2 CIRCUITS**	▸ **2 CIRCUITS**	Skipping (p. 164)	Skipping (p. 164)
Jump Squats (p. 174), 5–10 reps	Jump Squats (p. 174), 5–10 reps	High Skipping (p. 165)	High Skipping (p. 165)
V-Ups with Medball (p. 211), 5–10 reps	V-Ups (p. 211), 5–10 reps	Flat-Footed Marching (p. 166)	Flat-Footed Marching (p. 166)
Walking Lunges (p. 176), 5 lunges each side	Walking Lunges (p. 176), 5 lunges each side	Bounding (p. 127)	Bounding (p. 127)
30 sec. rest between exercises, 1 min. rest between circuits	30 sec. rest between exercises, 1 min. rest between circuits	High Knees (p. 167)	High Knees (p. 167)
		Straight-Leg Bounding (p. 171)	Straight-Leg Bounding (p. 171)
STRIDES		Quick Feet (p. 168)	Quick Feet (p. 168)
Strides (90%) (p. 182), 2 reps	Strides (90%) (p. 182), 2 reps	Butt Kicks (p. 170)	Butt Kicks (p. 170)
		After each drill, jog back to start, stride at 90% effort same distance as drill, walk back to start	After each drill, jog back to start, stride at 90% effort same distance as drill, walk back to start
Acceleration Exercises		**Maximum Velocity Exercises**	
Medball Push & Sprint (p. 131), 2 reps	Jump & Sprint (p. 128), 2 reps	Ankle Poppers (p. 178), 15 sec. each foot, 2 reps	Ankle Poppers (p. 178), 15 sec. each foot, 2 reps
Standing 5-Jump (p. 134), 2 sets of 5 jumps	Standing 5-Jump (p. 134), 2 sets of 5 jumps	Leg Lifts (p. 200), 2 sets of 25–30 reps	Leg Lifts (p. 200), 2 sets of 25–30 reps
Weight Sled Marching (p. 136), 15 yd., 2 reps	Stadium Steps Marching (p. 130), 15 sec., 2 reps	Heel Dips (p. 230), 2 sets of 15 reps each side	Heel Dips (p. 230), 2 sets of 15 reps each side
1–2 min. rest after each rep, 3 min. rest before Strength Circuit 2	1–2 min. rest after each rep, 3 min. rest before Strength Circuit 2	Depth Jumps (p. 173), 3 reps	Double-Leg Hops (p. 180), 3 reps
		2–3 min. rest after each rep	2–3 min. rest after each rep
Strength Circuit 2			
▸ **2 CIRCUITS**	▸ **2 CIRCUITS**		
Heel Dips (p. 230), 15 reps each side	Heel Dips (p. 230), 15 reps each side		
Leg Lifts (p. 200), 15–30 reps	Leg Lifts (p. 200), 15–30 reps		
Nordic Curls (p. 202), 8 reps (or Single-Leg Deadlifts (p. 208), 8 reps each side)	Nordic Curls (p. 202), 8 reps (or Single-Leg Deadlifts (p. 208), 8 reps each side)		
30 sec. rest between exercises, 1 min. rest between circuits	30 sec. rest between exercises, 1 min. rest between circuits		
FINAL EXERCISE		**FINAL EXERCISE**	
Resisted Run (p. 129), 2 × 10 sec.	Mountain Climbers (p. 203), 2 × 20 sec.	Hill Sprints and Stadium Steps (p. 130), 2 reps	Hill Sprints and Stadium Steps (p. 130), 2 reps
2 min. rest between reps	2 min. rest between reps	1 min. rest between reps	1 min. rest between reps

Build in 1–3 days of recovery between SpeedRunner sessions. The elective Speed Endurance day (see pages 97–102) should be followed by a day off.

WEEK 3

SESSION 1 ACCELERATION & STRENGTH		SESSION 2 MAXIMUM VELOCITY	
PROPS	**NO PROPS**	**PROPS**	**NO PROPS**
WARM-UP		**WARM-UP**	
Buildups 4-2-2 (p. 123)	Buildups 4-2-2 (p. 123)	Jogging (p. 122), 10–15 min.	Jogging (p. 122), 10–15 min.
Strength Circuit 1		**Technique Drills**	
▸ **2 CIRCUITS**	▸ **2 CIRCUITS**	Skipping (p. 164)	Skipping (p. 164)
Jump Squats with Weight (p. 175), *5–10 reps*	Jump Squats (p. 174), *5–10 reps*	High Skipping (p. 165)	High Skipping (p. 165)
Plank (p. 204), *30 sec.*	Plank (p. 204), *30 sec.*	Flat-Footed Marching (p. 166)	Flat-Footed Marching (p. 166)
Step-Downs (p. 229), *8–10 reps each side*	Step-Downs (p. 229), *8–10 reps each side*	Bounding (p. 127)	Bounding (p. 127)
30 sec. rest between exercises, 1 min. rest between circuits	**30 sec. rest between exercises, 1 min. rest between circuits**	High Knees (p. 167)	High Knees (p. 167)
		Straight-Leg Bounding (p. 171)	Straight-Leg Bounding (p. 171)
STRIDES		Quick Feet (p. 168)	Quick Feet (p. 168)
Strides (90%) (p. 182), *2 reps*	Strides (90%) (p. 182), *2 reps*	Quick Hops (p. 169)	Quick Hops (p. 169)
		Butt Kicks (p. 170)	Butt Kicks (p. 170)
		After each drill, jog back to start, stride at 90% effort same distance as drill, walk back to start	**After each drill, jog back to start, stride at 90% effort same distance as drill, walk back to start**
Acceleration Exercises		**Maximum Velocity Exercises**	
Weight Sled Push (p. 135), *10 yd., 2 reps*	3-Bounce & Run (p. 124), *2 reps*	Walking Lunges (p. 176), *5 lunges each side, 2 reps*	Walking Lunges (p. 176), *5 lunges each side, 2 reps*
3-Bounce & Run (p. 124), *2 reps*	Hill Sprints and Stadium Steps (p. 130), *2 reps*	Leg Lifts (p. 200), *2 sets of 25–30 reps*	Leg Lifts (p. 200), *2 sets of 25–30 reps*
Weight Sled Run (p. 138), *20 yd., 2 reps*	Downhill Sprints or 30-yd. sprints (95%) if no hill (p. 130), *2 reps*	Heel Dips (p. 230), *2 sets of 15–20 reps each side*	Heel Dips (p. 230), *2 sets of 15–20 reps each side*
1–2 min. rest after each rep, 3 min. rest before Strength Circuit 2	**1–2 min. rest after each rep, 3 min. rest before Strength Circuit 2**	Triple Hop on 1 Leg (p. 172), *2 reps each leg, alternating*	Triple Hop on 1 Leg (p. 172), *2 reps each leg, alternating*
		2–3 min. rest after each rep	**2–3 min. rest after each rep**
Strength Circuit 2			
▸ **2 CIRCUITS**	▸ **2 CIRCUITS**		
Heel Dips (p. 230), *15–20 reps each side*	Heel Dips (p. 230), *15–20 reps each side*		
Leg Lifts (p. 200), *15–30 reps*	Leg Lifts (p. 200), *15–30 reps*		
Nordic Curls (p. 202), *10 reps (or Single-Leg Deadlifts (p. 208), 10 reps each side)*	Nordic Curls (p. 202), *10 reps (or Single-Leg Deadlifts (p. 208), 10 reps each side)*		
30 sec. rest between exercises, 1 min. rest between circuits	**30 sec. rest between exercises, 1 min. rest between circuits**		
FINAL EXERCISE		**FINAL EXERCISE**	
Overhead Medball Throw (p. 220), *3 reps*	Bear Crawl (p. 196), *2 × 20 yd.*	Strides (95%) (p. 182), *65–75 yd., 2 reps*	Strides (95%) (p. 182), *65–75 yd., 2 reps*
1 min. rest between reps	**3 min. rest between reps**		

Build in 1–3 days of recovery between SpeedRunner sessions. The elective Speed Endurance day (see pages 97–102) should be followed by a day off.

WEEK 4

SESSION 1 **ACCELERATION & STRENGTH**		SESSION 2 **MAXIMUM VELOCITY**	
PROPS	**NO PROPS**	**PROPS**	**NO PROPS**
WARM-UP		**WARM-UP**	
Buildups 4-2-2 (p. 123)	Buildups 4-2-2 (p. 123)	Jogging (p. 122), *10–15 min.*	Jogging (p. 122), *10–15 min.*
Strength Circuit 1		**Technique Drills**	
▸ **2 CIRCUITS** Jump Squats with Weight (p. 175), *5–10 reps* V-Ups with Medball (p. 211), *5–10 reps* Walking Lunges (p. 176), *5 lunges each side* **30 sec. rest between exercises, 1 min. rest between circuits**	▸ **2 CIRCUITS** Jump Squats (p. 174), *5–10 reps* V-Ups (p. 211), *5–10 reps* Walking Lunges (p. 176), *5 lunges each side* **30 sec. rest between exercises, 1 min. rest between circuits**	Skipping (p. 164) High Skipping (p. 165) Flat-Footed Marching (p. 166) Bounding (p. 127) High Knees (p. 167) Straight-Leg Bounding (p. 171) Quick Feet (p. 168) Quick Hops (p. 169) Butt Kicks (p. 170)	Skipping (p. 164) High Skipping (p. 165) Flat-Footed Marching (p. 166) Bounding (p. 127) High Knees (p. 167) Straight-Leg Bounding (p. 171) Quick Feet (p. 168) Quick Hops (p. 169) Butt Kicks (p. 170)
STRIDES		After each drill, jog back to start, stride at 90% effort same distance as drill, walk back to start	After each drill, jog back to start, stride at 90% effort same distance as drill, walk back to start
Strides (90%) (p. 182), *2 reps*	Strides (90%) (p. 182), *2 reps*		
Acceleration Exercises		**Maximum Velocity Exercises**	
Weight Sled Push (p. 135), *10–20 yd., 2 reps* 3-Point Stance & Sprint (p. 126), *2 reps* Weight Sled Run (p. 138), *20 yd., 2 reps* **1–2 min. rest after each rep, 3 min. rest before Strength Circuit 2**	3-Point Stance & Sprint (p. 126), *2 reps* Stadium Steps Marching (p. 137), *15 sec., 2 reps* Downhill Sprints or 30-yd. sprints (95%) if no hill (p. 130), *2 reps* **1–2 min. rest after each rep, 3 min. rest before Strength Circuit 2**	Ankle Poppers (p. 178), *15 sec. each foot, 2 reps* Leg Lifts (p. 200), *2 sets of 25–30 reps* Heel Dips (p. 230), *2 sets of 15–20 reps each side* Depth Jumps (p. 173), *3 reps* **2–3 min. rest after each rep**	Ankle Poppers (p. 178), *15 sec. each foot, 2 reps* Leg Lifts (p. 200), *2 sets of 25–30 reps* Heel Dips (p. 230), *2 sets of 15–20 reps each side* Double-Leg Hops (p. 180), *3 reps* or Single-Leg Hops (if you're ready) (p. 181), *1–2 reps each leg* **2–3 min. rest after each rep**
Strength Circuit 2			
▸ **2 CIRCUITS** Heel Dips (p. 230), *15–20 reps each side* Leg Lifts (p. 200), *15–30 reps* Nordic Curls (p. 202), *10 reps* (or Single-Leg Deadlifts (p. 208), *10 reps each side*) **30 sec. rest between exercises, 1 min. rest between circuits**	▸ **2 CIRCUITS** Heel Dips (p. 230), *15–20 reps each side* Leg Lifts (p. 200), *15–30 reps* Nordic Curls (p. 202), *10 reps* (or Single-Leg Deadlifts (p. 208), *10 reps each side*) **30 sec. rest between exercises, 1 min. rest between circuits**		
FINAL EXERCISE		**FINAL EXERCISE**	
Resisted Run (p. 129), *2 × 10 sec.* **2 min. rest between reps**	Mountain Climbers (p. 203), *2 × 20 sec.* **2 min. rest between reps**	Hill Sprints and Stadium Steps (p. 130), *4 reps* **1 min. rest between reps**	Hill Sprints and Stadium Steps (p. 130), *4 reps* **1 min. rest between reps**

Build in 1–3 days of recovery between SpeedRunner sessions. The elective Speed Endurance day (see pages 97–102) should be followed by a day off.

DISTANCE RUNNER
ONCE-PER-WEEK SCHEDULE

✔ Four weeks

✔ One session per week

✔ Treat as a hard day, to be preceded and followed by an easy day of training

A sample week of the Distance Runner schedule might look like this:

MON.	TUES.	WED.	THURS.	FRI.	SAT.	SUN.
Intervals/ tempo		Speed work	Easy training	**Session** Drills & Speed	Easy training	Long run

250

WEEK 1	WEEK 2	WEEK 3	WEEK 4
WARM-UP			
Jogging (p. 122), *10–15 min.*	Jogging (p. 122), *10–15 min.*	Jogging (p. 122), *10–15 min.*	Jogging (p. 122), *10–15 min.*
Technique Drills			
Skipping (p. 164) High Skipping (p. 165) Flat-Footed Marching (p. 166) High Knees (p. 167) Quick Feet (p. 168) Butt Kicks (p. 170) **After each drill, jog back to start, stride at 90% effort same distance as drill, walk back to start**	Skipping (p. 164) High Skipping (p. 165) Flat-Footed Marching (p. 166) Bounding (p. 127) High Knees (p. 167) Quick Feet (p. 168) Butt Kicks (p. 170) **After each drill, jog back to start, stride at 90% effort same distance as drill, walk back to start**	Skipping (p. 164) High Skipping (p. 165) Flat-Footed Marching (p. 166) Bounding (p. 127) High Knees (p. 167) Quick Feet (p. 168) Quick Hops (p. 169) Butt Kicks (p. 170) **After each drill, jog back to start, stride at 90% effort same distance as drill, walk back to start**	Skipping (p. 164) High Skipping (p. 165) Flat-Footed Marching (p. 166) Bounding (p. 127) High Knees (p. 167) Quick Feet (p. 168) Quick Hops (p. 169) Butt Kicks (p. 170) **After each drill, jog back to start, stride at 90% effort same distance as drill, walk back to start**
Speed Exercises			
Standing Starts (forward sprints only) (p. 133), *1 rep each leg* Hill Sprints and Stadium Steps (p. 130), *2 reps* **1–2 min. rest after each rep, 3 min. rest before strength circuit**	Triple Hop on 1 Leg (p. 172), *1 rep each leg* Hill Sprints and Stadium Steps (p. 130), *2 reps* **1–2 min. rest after each rep, 3 min. rest before strength circuit**	Standing Starts (forward sprints only) (p. 133), *1 rep each leg* Hill Sprints and Stadium Steps (p. 130), *4 reps* **1–2 min. rest after each rep, 3 min. rest before strength circuit**	Triple Hop on 1 Leg (p. 172), *1 rep each leg* Hill Sprints and Stadium Steps (p. 130), *4 reps* **1–2 min. rest after each rep, 3 min. rest before strength circuit**
Strength Circuit			
▶ **2 CIRCUITS**	▶ **2 CIRCUITS**	▶ **2 CIRCUITS**	▶ **2 CIRCUITS**
Heel Dips (p. 230), *10 reps each side* Leg Lifts (p. 200), *10–20 reps* Nordic Curls (p. 202), *5 reps* (or Single-Leg Deadlifts (p. 208), *5 reps each side*) **30 sec. rest between exercises, 1 min. rest between circuits**	Heel Dips (p. 230), *15 reps each side* Leg Lifts (p. 200), *15–30 reps* Nordic Curls (p. 202), *8 reps* (or Single-Leg Deadlifts (p. 208), *8 reps each side*) **30 sec. rest between exercises, 1 min. rest between circuits**	Heel Dips (p. 230), *15–20 reps each side* Leg Lifts (p. 200), *15–30 reps* Nordic Curls (p. 202), *10 reps* (or Single-Leg Deadlifts (p. 208), *10 reps each side*) **30 sec. rest between exercises, 1 min. rest between circuits**	Heel Dips (p. 230), *15–20 reps each side* Leg Lifts (p. 200), *15–30 reps* Nordic Curls (p. 202), *10 reps* (or Single-Leg Deadlifts (p. 208), *10 reps each side*) **30 sec. rest between exercises, 1 min. rest between circuits**

Since this once-a-week speed day is a hard session, build in easy days of training before and after.

SOLO SESSIONS

✔ Two workouts (two days of training) per fitness target

✔ No more than three sessions per week

✔ One to three recovery days between sessions

✔ Perform only on days when you have no other training scheduled or your other athletic activity is low-intensity

A sample week of the Solo Session schedule might look like this:

MON.	TUES.	WED.	THURS.	FRI.	SAT.	SUN.
Session 1 Acceleration	Recovery	Recovery	**Session 2** Acceleration	Recovery		

ACCELERATION

SESSION 1		SESSION 2	
PROPS	**NO PROPS**	**PROPS**	**NO PROPS**
WARM-UP		**WARM-UP**	
Buildups 4-2-2 (p. 123)	Buildups 4-2-2 (p. 123)	Buildups 4-2-2 (p. 123)	Buildups 4-2-2 (p. 123)
Strength Circuit		**Strength Circuit**	
▸ **2 CIRCUITS** Jump Squats with Weight (p. 175), *5–10 reps* Leg Lifts (p. 200), *20 reps* Battle Ropes (p. 218), *30 sec.* **30 sec. rest between exercises, 1 min. rest between circuits**	▸ **2 CIRCUITS** Jump Squats (p. 174), *5–10 reps* Leg Lifts (p. 200), *20 reps* Plyo Push-Ups (p. 224), *5–10 reps* **30 sec. rest between exercises, 1 min. rest between circuits**	▸ **2 CIRCUITS** Single-Leg Squat (p. 207), *5–10 reps each leg* V-Ups with Medball (p. 211), *10 reps* Battle Ropes (p. 218), *30 sec.* **30 sec. rest between exercises, 1 min. rest between circuits**	▸ **2 CIRCUITS** Single-Leg Squat (p. 207), *5–10 reps each leg* V-Ups (p. 211), *10 reps* Plyo Push-Ups (p. 224), *5–10 reps* **30 sec. rest between exercises, 1 min. rest between circuits**
STRIDES		**STRIDES**	
Strides (90%) (p. 182), *2 reps*	Strides (90%) (p. 182), *2 reps*	Strides (90%) (p. 182), *2 reps*	Strides (90%) (p. 182), *2 reps*
Acceleration Exercises		**Acceleration Exercises**	
Weight Sled Push (p. 135), *10 yd., 2 reps* Weight Sled Run (p. 138), *20 yd., 2 reps* Kneeling Partner Medball Twist (p. 213), *30 sec., 2 reps* or Windshield Wipers (p. 212), *2 sets of 10 reps each side* Hip Thrusts (with bench) (p. 214), *2 sets of 5–10 reps* Mountain Climbers (p. 203), *20 sec., 2 reps* Overhead Medball Throw (p. 220), *3 reps* Strides (90%) (p. 182), *2 reps* **1–2 min. rest after each rep**	Stadium Steps Marching (p. 130), *15 sec., 2 reps* or 3-Bounce & Run (p. 124), *2 reps* Hill Sprints and Stadium Steps (p. 130), *2 reps* Kneeling Partner Medball Twist (p. 213), *30 sec., 2 reps* or Windshield Wipers (p. 212), *2 sets of 10 reps each side* Hip Thrusts (ground level) (p. 215), *5–10 reps* Mountain Climbers (p. 203), *20 sec., 2 reps* Mini-Suicides (p. 151), *2 reps* Strides (90%) (p. 182), *2 reps* **1–2 min. rest after each rep**	Medball Push & Sprint (p. 131), *2 reps* Resisted Run (p. 129), *10 sec., 2 reps* Plank (p. 204), *1 rep of 30–60 sec.* Standing 5-Jump (p. 134), *2 sets of 5 jumps* Walking Lunges (p. 176), *5 lunges each side, 2 reps* 3-Point Stance & Sprint (p. 126), *2 reps* Hill Sprints and Stadium Steps (p. 130), *2 reps* **1–2 min. rest after each rep**	Jump & Sprint (p. 128), *2 reps* Standing Starts (forward sprints only) (p. 133), *2 sets* or Mountain Climbers (p. 203), *20 sec., 2 reps* Plank (p. 204), *1 rep of 30–60 sec.* Standing 5-Jump (p. 134), *2 sets of 5 jumps* Walking Lunges (p. 176), *5 lunges each side, 2 reps* 3-Point Stance & Sprint (p. 126), *2 reps* Hill Sprints and Stadium Steps (p. 130), *2 reps* **1–2 min. rest after each rep**

Build in 1–3 days of recovery between sessions. Perform only on days when your other athletic activity is low-intensity.

MAXIMUM VELOCITY

SESSION 1		SESSION 2	
PROPS	**NO PROPS**	**PROPS**	**NO PROPS**
WARM-UP		**WARM-UP**	
Jogging (p. 122), 10–15 min.	Jogging (p. 122), 10–15 min.	Jogging (p. 122), 10–15 min.	Jogging (p. 122), 10–15 min.
Technique Drills		**Technique Drills**	
Skipping (p. 164)	Skipping (p. 164)	Skipping (p. 164)	Skipping (p. 164)
High Skipping (p. 165)	High Skipping (p. 165)	High Skipping (p. 165)	High Skipping (p. 165)
Flat-Footed Marching (p. 166)	Flat-Footed Marching (p. 166)	Flat-Footed Marching (p. 166)	Flat-Footed Marching (p. 166)
Bounding (p. 127)	Bounding (p. 127)	Bounding (p. 127)	Bounding (p. 127)
High Knees (p. 167)	High Knees (p. 167)	High Knees (p. 167)	High Knees (p. 167)
Quick Feet (p. 168)	Quick Feet (p. 168)	Quick Feet (p. 168)	Quick Feet (p. 168)
Quick Hops (p. 169)	Quick Hops (p. 169)	Quick Hops (p. 169)	Quick Hops (p. 169)
Butt Kicks (p. 170)	Butt Kicks (p. 170)	Butt Kicks (p. 170)	Butt Kicks (p. 170)
After each drill, jog back to start, stride at 90% effort same distance as drill, walk back to start	**After each drill, jog back to start, stride at 90% effort same distance as drill, walk back to start**	**After each drill, jog back to start, stride at 90% effort same distance as drill, walk back to start**	**After each drill, jog back to start, stride at 90% effort same distance as drill, walk back to start**
Maximum Velocity Exercises		**Maximum Velocity Exercises**	
Ankle Poppers (p. 178), *15 sec. each foot, 2 reps*	Ankle Poppers (p. 178), *15 sec. each foot, 2 reps*	Weighted Ankle Poppers (p. 179), *30 sec. each foot, 2 reps*	Weighted Ankle Poppers (use prop swap) (p. 179), *30 sec. each foot, 2 reps*
Fire Hydrant (p. 199), *2 sets of 10 reps each side*	Fire Hydrant (p. 199), *2 sets of 10 reps each side*	Step-Downs (p. 229), *2 sets of 10 reps each side*	Step-Downs (p. 229), *2 sets of 10 reps each side*
Nordic Curls (p. 202), *2 sets of 10 reps [or Single-Leg Deadlifts (p. 208), 2 sets of 10 reps each side]*	Nordic Curls (p. 202), *2 sets of 10 reps [or Single-Leg Deadlifts (p. 208), 2 sets of 10 reps each side]*	Single-Leg Deadlifts (p. 208), *2 sets of 10 reps each side*	Single-Leg Deadlifts (p. 208), *2 sets of 10 reps each side*
Depth Jumps (p. 173), *2 reps*	Double-Leg Hops (p. 180), *2 reps*	Triple Hop on 1 Leg (p. 172), *2 reps each leg*	Triple Hop on 1 Leg (p. 172), *2 reps each leg*
Gassers 30/30 (p. 183), *2 reps*	Gassers 30/30 (p. 183), *2 reps*	40-Yard Dash (p. 186), *1 rep*	40-Yard Dash (p. 186), *1 rep*
1–2 min. rest after each rep	**1–2 min. rest after each rep**	**1–2 min. rest after each rep**	**1–2 min. rest after each rep**

Build in 1–3 days of recovery between sessions. Perform only on days when your other athletic activity is low-intensity.

WHOLE-BODY STRENGTH

SESSION 1		SESSION 2	
PROPS	**NO PROPS**	**PROPS**	**NO PROPS**
WARM-UP		**WARM-UP**	
Buildups 4-2-2 (p. 123)	Buildups 4-2-2 (p. 123)	Buildups 4-2-2 (p. 123)	Buildups 4-2-2 (p. 123)
Strength Circuit		**Strength Circuit**	
▸ **2 CIRCUITS** Jump Squats with Weight (p. 175), *5–10 reps* V-Ups with Medball (p. 211), *10 reps* Plyo Push-Ups (p. 224), *5–10 reps* 30 sec. rest between exercises, 1 min. rest between circuits	▸ **2 CIRCUITS** Jump Squats (p. 174), *5–10 reps* V-Ups (p. 211), *10 reps* Plyo Push-Ups (p. 224), *5–10 reps* 30 sec. rest between exercises, 1 min. rest between circuits	▸ **2 CIRCUITS** Step-Ups (p. 228), *5–10 reps each leg* Kneeling Partner Medball Twist (p. 213), *30 sec.* or Windshield Wipers (p. 212), *10 reps each side* Battle Ropes (p. 218), *30 sec.* 30 sec. rest between exercises, 1 min. rest between circuits	▸ **2 CIRCUITS** Step-Ups (p. 228), *5–10 reps each leg* Kneeling Partner Medball Twist (p. 213), *30 sec.* or Windshield Wipers (p. 212), *10 reps each side* Plyo Push-Ups (p. 224), *5–10 reps* 30 sec. rest between exercises, 1 min. rest between circuits
STRIDES		**STRIDES**	
Strides (90%) (p. 182), *2 reps*	Strides (90%) (p. 182), *2 reps*	Strides (90%) (p. 182), *2 reps*	Strides (90%) (p. 182), *2 reps*
Whole-Body Exercises		**Whole-Body Exercises**	
Weight Sled Marching (p. 136), *15 yd., 2 reps* Weight Sled Crossover (p. 160), *10 yd., 2 reps, switch direction for 2nd rep* Hip Thrusts (with bench) (p. 214), *2 sets of 5–10 reps* Plank (p. 204), *30–60 sec., 2 reps* Mountain Climbers (p. 203), *20 sec., 2 reps* Overhead Medball Throw (p. 220), *3 reps* Strides (90%) (p. 182), *2 reps* 1–2 min. rest after each rep	Stadium Steps Marching (p. 137), *15 sec., 2 reps* Stadium Crossover Steps (p. 161), *5–10 steps, 2 reps, reverse front/back leg for 2nd rep* Hip Thrusts (ground level) (p. 215), *2 sets of 5–10 reps* Plank (p. 204), *30–60 sec., 2 reps* Mountain Climbers (p. 203), *20 sec., 2 reps* Crab Walk (p. 197), *2 sets of 2 × 10 yd.* Strides (90%) (p. 182), *2 reps* 1–2 min. rest after each rep	Crab Walk (p. 197), *10 yd., 2 reps* Marching Bridge (p. 201), *2 sets of 5–10 reps each leg* Bear Crawl (p. 196), *20 yd., 2 reps* Plank Rotations (p. 205), *2 sets of 5–10 reps each side* Monster Walk (p. 226), *2 reps* Tug Rope with Weight Sled or Free Weight (p. 217), *2 reps* Strides (90%) (p. 182), *2 reps* 1–2 min. rest after each rep	Crab Walk (p. 197), *10 yd., 2 reps* Marching Bridge (p. 201), *2 sets of 5–10 reps each leg* Bear Crawl (p. 196), *20 yd., 2 reps* Plank Rotations (p. 205), *2 sets of 5–10 reps each side* Side Leg Lifts (p. 206), *2 sets of 10 reps each leg* Pull-Ups (p. 217), *2 sets of maximum pull-up reps* Strides (90%) (p. 182), *2 reps* 1–2 min. rest after each rep

Build in 1–3 days of recovery between sessions. Perform only on days when your other athletic activity is low-intensity.

CORE MUSCLES & HIPS

	SESSION 1		SESSION 2	
PROPS	**NO PROPS**	**PROPS**	**NO PROPS**
WARM-UP		**WARM-UP**	
Jogging (p. 122), *12–15 min.*	Jogging (p. 122), *12–15 min.*	Jogging (p. 122), *12–15 min.*	Jogging (p. 122), *12–15 min.*
Strength Circuit		**Strength Circuit**	
▸ **2 CIRCUITS**	▸ **2 CIRCUITS**	▸ **2 CIRCUITS**	▸ **2 CIRCUITS**
Russian Oblique Twist (p. 225), *10 reps each side* Fire Hydrants (p. 199), *5–10 reps each side* Leg Lifts (p. 200), *15–30 reps* 30 sec. rest between exercises, 1 min. rest between circuits	Russian Oblique Twist (p. 225), *10 reps each side* Fire Hydrants (p. 199), *5–10 reps each side* Leg Lifts (p. 200), *15–30 reps* 30 sec. rest between exercises, 1 min. rest between circuits	Kneeling Partner Medball Twist (p. 213), *30 sec.* or Windshield Wipers (p. 212), *10 reps each side* Fire Hydrants (p. 199), *5–10 reps each side* V-Ups with Medball (p. 211), *10 reps* 30 sec. rest between exercises, 1 min. rest between circuits	Kneeling Partner Medball Twist (p. 213), *30 sec.* or Windshield Wipers (p. 212), *10 reps each side* Fire Hydrants (p. 199), *5–10 reps each side* V-Ups (p. 211), *10 reps* 30 sec. rest between exercises, 1 min. rest between circuits
STRIDES		**STRIDES**	
Strides (90%) (p. 182), *2 reps*	Strides (90%) (p. 182), *2 reps*	Strides (90%) (p. 182), *2 reps*	Strides (90%) (p. 182), *2 reps*
Core & Hip Exercises		**Core & Hip Exercises**	
Side Steps with Resistance Band (p. 227), *10 steps each direction, 2 reps* Plank (p. 204), *30–60 sec., 2 reps* Weight Sled Crossover (p. 160), *10 yd., 2 reps, switch direction for 2nd rep* Marching Bridge (p. 201), *2 sets of 5–10 reps each leg* Bird Dogs (p. 198), *2 sets of 5–10 reps each side, alternating* or Superman/Superwoman Plank (p. 210), *2 sets of 5–10 reps each side, alternating* Hip Thrusts (with bench) (p. 214), *2 sets of 5–10 reps* Strides (90%) (p. 182), *2 reps* 1–2 min. rest after each rep	Side Leg Lifts (p. 206), *2 sets of 10 reps each side* Plank (p. 204), *30–60 sec., 2 reps* Stadium Crossover Steps (p. 161), *5–10 steps, 2 reps, reverse front/back leg for 2nd rep* Marching Bridge (p. 201), *2 sets of 5–10 reps each leg* Bird Dogs (p. 198), *2 sets of 5–10 reps each side, alternating* or Superman/Superwoman Plank (p. 210), *2 sets of 5–10 reps each side, alternating* Hip Thrusts (ground level) (p. 215), *2 sets of 5–10 reps* Strides (90%) (p. 182), *2 reps* 1–2 min. rest after each rep	Side Steps (Quick) (p. 149), *15–20 yd. each direction, 2 reps* Plank Rotations (p. 205), *2 sets of 5–10 reps each side* Lunge Clock (p. 216), *1 revolution each direction* Marching Bridge (p. 201), *2 sets of 5–10 reps each leg* Bird Dogs (p. 198), *2 sets of 5–10 reps each side, alternating* or Superman/Superwoman Plank (p. 210), *2 sets of 5–10 reps each side, alternating* Mountain Climbers (p. 203), *20 sec., 2 reps* Strides (90%) (p. 182), *2 reps* 1–2 min. rest after each rep	Side Steps (Quick) (p. 149), *15–20 yd. each direction, 2 reps* Plank Rotations (p. 205), *2 sets of 5–10 reps each side* Lunge Clock (p. 216), *1 revolution each direction* Marching Bridge (p. 201), *2 sets of 5–10 reps each leg* Bird Dogs (p. 198), *2 sets of 5–10 reps each side, alternating* or Superman/Superwoman Plank (p. 210), *2 sets of 5–10 reps each side, alternating* Mountain Climbers (p. 203), *20 sec., 2 reps* Strides (90%) (p. 182), *2 reps* 1–2 min. rest after each rep

Build in 1–3 days of recovery between sessions. Perform only on days when your other athletic activity is low-intensity.

INJURY PREVENTION

SESSION

PROPS	NO PROPS
WARM-UP	
Jogging (p. 122), *10–15 min.*	Jogging (p. 122), *10–15 min.*

Strength Circuit

▶ **2 CIRCUITS**	▶ **2 CIRCUITS**
Air Squats (p. 194), *10 reps*	Air Squats (p. 194), *10 reps*
Step-Ups (p. 228), *10 reps each leg*	Step-Ups (p. 228), *10 reps each leg*
Leg Lifts (p. 200), *20 reps*	Leg Lifts (p. 200), *20 reps*
30 sec. rest between exercises, 1 min. rest between circuits	**30 sec. rest between exercises, 1 min. rest between circuits**

STRIDES	
Strides (90%) (p. 182), *2 reps*	Strides (90%) (p. 182), *2 reps*

Injury-Prevention Exercises

Heel Dips (p. 230), *2 sets of 20 reps each side*	Heel Dips (p. 230), *2 sets of 20 reps each side*
Single-Leg Deadlifts (p. 208), *2 sets of 10 reps each side*	Single-Leg Deadlifts (p. 208), *2 sets of 10 reps each side*
Nordic Curls (p. 202), *2 sets of 10 reps*	Nordic Curls (p. 202), *2 sets of 10 reps (if you can't do these, skip to next exercise)*
Step-Downs (p. 229), *2 sets of 10 reps each side*	Step-Downs (p. 229), *2 sets of 10 reps each side*
Side Steps with Resistance Band (p. 227), *10 steps each direction, 2 reps*	Side Leg Lifts (p. 206), *2 sets of 10 reps each leg*
Monster Walk (p. 226), *10 steps each leg, 2 reps*	Side Steps (Quick) (p. 149), *15 yd., 2 reps each direction*
Backward Running (p. 150), *20 yd., 2 reps*	Backward Running (p. 150), *20 yd., 2 reps*
1–2 min. rest after each rep	**1–2 min. rest after each rep**

Perform only on days when your other athletic activity is low-intensity.

METRICS TEST

Track your progress by performing the four basic metrics, in order. You can complete these tests before and after the SpeedRunner program.

PRE-SPEEDRUNNER PROGRAM

WARM-UP		

Jogging (p. 122), *10–15 min.*
Strides (90%) (p. 182), *4 reps*
3 min. rest after strides

Metrics Tests		
	Results	Notes
40-Yard Dash (p. 186)		
Standing Broad Jump (p. 187)		
20-Yard Shuttle (p. 188)		
3-Cone Drill (p. 190)		

3–10 min. rest between tests

ADDITIONAL TESTS		
	Results	Notes
Vertical Leap		
Your Choice		

3–10 min. rest between tests

POST-SPEEDRUNNER PROGRAM

WARM-UP

Jogging (p. 122), *10–15 min.*
Strides (90%) (p. 182), *4 reps*
3 min. rest after strides

Metrics Tests		
	Results	Notes
40-Yard Dash (p. 186)		
Standing Broad Jump (p. 187)		
20-Yard Shuttle (p. 188)		
3-Cone Drill (p. 190)		

3–10 min. rest between tests

ADDITIONAL TESTS		
	Results	Notes
Vertical Leap		
Your Choice		

3–10 min. rest between tests

PROPS, NO-PROP OPTIONS, AND PROP SWAPS

Prop exercises are listed with "No-Props Alternatives" (if available), with additional information on "prop swaps." Prop swaps are everyday items you can use to replace a prop, making it possible to perform the "Props" version of the exercise even if you don't have access to the designated prop.

PROPS EXERCISES	PROPS	NO-PROPS ALTERNATIVE(S)	PROP SWAP
Agility Ladder 1-Legged Hops	Agility ladder	Agility 1-Legged Hops × 10 reps (12–14 inches per hop)	Markers every 12–24 inches to create landing spaces (cards, coasters, coins, or other small, flat objects; avoid using raised objects)
Agility Ladder 2-Legged Hops	Agility ladder	Agility 2-Legged Hops × 10 reps (12–24 inches per hop)	Markers every 12–24 inches to create landing spaces (cards, coasters, coins, or other small, flat objects; avoid using raised objects)
Agility Ladder 3 Quick Steps	Agility ladder	3-Step, 1-Step	Markers every 12–24 inches to create landing spaces (cards, coasters, coins, or other small, flat objects; avoid using raised objects)
Agility Ladder Ickey Shuffle	Agility ladder	Use prop swap	Marked line on field or create a line using markers (paper plates, shoes, small stones, cards, coasters, etc.) or do the exercise without markers
Agility Ladder Step In 'n' Out	Agility ladder	Step Back 'n' Forth Drill	No prop swap; do no-prop alternative
Air Squats with Medball	Medball	Use prop swap	Any ball or lightweight object (e.g., light dumbbell) that you can hold while maintaining balance
Battle Ropes	Battle ropes	Push-Ups, Plyo Push-Ups, Bear Crawl, Crab Walk	No prop swap; do no-prop alternative

>>

PROPS EXERCISES	PROPS	NO-PROPS ALTERNATIVE(S)	PROP SWAP
Cone Drills (all)	Cones	Use prop swap	Paper plates, shoes, small stones, cards, coasters, etc.
Depth Jump	Plyo box	Double-Leg Hops, Single-Leg Hops	Bench, bottom bleacher, any short platform that is 12–30 inches in height
Heel Dips	Short platform	Use prop swap or flat surface	Steps, bleachers, curb, etc.
Hip Thrust	Bench	Do at ground level	No prop swap; do no-prop alternative
Jump Squats with Weight	Weight vest or dumbbells	Jump Squats	No prop swap; do no-prop alternative
Kneeling Partner Medball Twist	Medball	Use prop swap	Any ball or lightweight object (e.g., light dumbbell)
Medball Push & Sprint	Medball	Jump & Sprint	No prop swap; do alternate exercise
Medball Push from Knees	Medball	Plyo Push-Ups	No prop swap; do alternate exercise
Mini-Suicides	Cones	Use prop swap	Marked lines on field/create lines using markers (paper plates, shoes, small stones, cards, coasters, etc.)
Monster Walk	Resistance band	Side Leg Lifts	No prop swap; do no-prop alternative
Nordic Curls	Partner or ankle restraint of some kind	Single-Leg Deadlift (but try to do Nordic Curls, as it's the best hamstring exercise)	Furniture (e.g., secure feet under bed) or any other object under which you can pin your feet and ankles
Overhead Medball Throw	Medball	None	No prop swap
Push-Ups with Medball	Medball	Use prop swap	Any ball or a short platform (you'll get less balance work with a platform than a ball)
Resisted Run	Resistance harness and tether	Mountain Climbers, Standing Starts (forward sprints only), Hill Sprints & Stadium Steps	No prop swap; do no-prop alternative
Russian Oblique Twist with Medball	Medball	Use prop swap	Any ball or lightweight object (e.g., light dumbbell)
Side Steps with Resistance Band	Resistance band	Side Leg Lifts/ Side Steps (Quick)	No prop swap available (if you own ankle weights, you can perform side steps with those and get a similar stimulus)

>>

PROPS EXERCISES	PROPS	NO-PROPS ALTERNATIVE(S)	PROP SWAP
Single-Leg Deadlift with Medball or Dumbbell	Medball or dumbbell	Use prop swap	Any ball or lightweight object
Single-Leg Squat from a Seated Position	Plyo box, chair	Use prop swap or perform without prop	Chair (not a folding chair due to balance issues) or other platform (must be as high as the lowest point of your squat)
Standing Broad Jump	Standing broad jump mat	Use prop swap	Measuring tape (or other makeshift measuring strategy)
Step-Downs	Bench or short platform	Use prop swap	Steps, bleachers, curb, etc.
Step-Ups	Bench or short platform	Use prop swap	Steps, bleachers, etc.
Tug Rope with Weight Sled or Free Weight	Battle rope and weight sled and/or weights	Pull-Ups	No prop swap; do no-prop alternative
V-Ups with Medball	Medball	Use prop swap	Any ball or lightweight object
Walking Lunges (with added weight)	Weight vest or dumbbells	Use prop swap	Two 1-gallon milk jugs filled with water (1 quart of water = 2 pounds), 1 held in each hand
Weight Sled Crossover	Weight sled	Crossover steps	Stadium steps or any flight of steps
Weight Sled Marching	Weight sled	Stadium Steps (Marching), Jump Squats	Stadium steps or any flight of steps
Weight Sled Push	Weight sled	Stadium Steps (Marching), 3-Point Stance & Sprint, 3-Bounce & Run, Hill Sprints & Stadium Steps, Jump Squats	Hill or stadium steps
Weight Sled Run	Weight sled	Downhill Sprints/ Hill Sprints or Stadium Steps (5 seconds total)	Hill or stadium steps
Weighted Ankle Poppers	Weight vest or dumbbells	Use prop swap or perform without weight	Two 1-gallon milk jugs filled with water (1 quart of water = 2 pounds), 1 held in each hand

ACKNOWLEDGMENTS

Unlike the athletes it seeks to inspire and mold, *SpeedRunner* did not explode off the start line and accelerate directly into final draft form. Instead, it is the end product of an extended and arduous team effort.

Thanks first to Casey Blaine, my editor, for her patience, skill, and commitment to this project—to the point of spending three days in Southern California to lend her expertise to the book's photo shoot. Thanks also to Vicki Hopewell, creative director for the book, and Kara Mannix, marketing and sales, both of whom also helped oversee that shoot. And to project editor Andy Read and Dave Trendler, marketing and sales, as well as to Christine Bucher, the book's copy editor.

Next, thanks to my agent, Thomas Flannery Jr., and to David Vigliano and everyone else at AGI Vigliano Literary.

Thanks to the book's models for their patience, professionalism, and efforts above and beyond (in scorching, near-100 degree temps): Sean Magill, Leilani Rios, and Telanto Harvey.

And thanks to Michael P. Parkinson, PT, for his physiological expertise and insights into the running gait cycle. Mike has cheerfully volunteered his time and know-how to every book I've written, a turn of events I couldn't have predicted four decades ago when we were archrivals in high school track.

This book represents the efforts, experience, scientific inquiry, and innovations of literally hundreds of coaches, athletes, exercise physiologists, and others who've contributed to the advancement of sports training methods and performance. Listing them all would require an additional chapter, so I'd like to thank them en masse—and to apologize if I've incorrectly interpreted any of their conclusions or recommendations. Any errors are mine.

Finally, I'd like to thank Diana Hernandez for once again lending her photographic talent to one of my running projects. I realized early on as a running-writer that a good photo was worth much more than a thousand of my words, and from *Runner's World* features shot in the snow and cold to this book's three-day shoot in the Southern California heat, Diana has always provided the types of photos that engage an audience—and even inspire some of them to read the accompanying text.

SELECTED BIBLIOGRAPHY

The following is a partial list of the many studies, reviews, and resources I consulted in preparation of the SpeedRunner program and book. It is by no means a complete list of references but a collection of many I find useful for the curious reader.

Chapter 1

Karni, Avi, Gundela Meyer, Christine Rey-Hipolito, Peter Jezzard, Michelle M. Adams, Robert Turner, and Lesli. G. Ungerleider. "The Acquisition of Skilled Motor Performance: Fast and Slow Experience-Driven Changes in Primary Motor Cortex." *Proceedings of the National Academy of Sciences* 95 no. 3 (1998): 861–68. doi:10.1073/pnas.95.3.861.

Ranganathan, Rajiv, Chandramouli Krishnan, Yasin Y. Dhaher, and William Z. Rymer. "Learning New Gait Patterns: Exploratory Muscle Activity during Motor Learning Is Not Predicted by Motor Modules." *Journal of Biomechanics* 49 no. 5 (2016): 718–25. doi:10.1016/j.jbiomech.2016.02.006.

"Research Reports: Participation Reports." 2017. *Sports & Fitness Industry Association.* https://www.sfia .org/reports/participation/.

Rumpf, Michael C., John B. Cronin, Ikhwan N. Mohamad, Sharil Mohamad, Jon L. Oliver, and Michael G. Hughes. "The Effect of Resisted Sprint Training on Maximum Sprint Kinetics and Kinematics in Youth." *European Journal of Sport Science* 15 no. 5 (2015): 374–81. doi:10.1080/17461391.2014.955125.

Sawers, Andrew, Jessica L. Allen, and Lena H. Ting. "Long-Term Training Modifies the Modular Structure and Organization of Walking Balance Control." *Journal of Neurophysiology* 114 no. 6 (2015): 3359–73. http://jn.physiology.org/content/early/2015/10/09/jn.00758.2015.

Walker, Owen. "Peak Height Velocity (PHV) | Science for Sport." *Science for Sport.* 2016. https://www .scienceforsport.com/peak-height-velocity.

Chapter 2

Adolph, Karen E., Whitney G. Cole, Meghana Komati, Jessie S. Garciaguirre, Daryaneh Badaly, Jesse M. Lingeman, Gladys L. Y. Chan, and Rachel B. Sotsky. "How Do You Learn to Walk? Thousands of Steps and Dozens of Falls per Day." *Psychological Science* 23 no. 11 (2012): 1387–94. doi:10.1177/0956797612446346.

Dicharry, Jay. "Kinematics and Kinetics of Gait: From Lab to Clinic." *Clinics in Sports Medicine* 29 no. 3 (2010): 347–64. doi:10.1016/j.csm.2010.03.013.

Lee, Jimson. "Triple Extension, Vertical Displacement, Stride Length, and Ground Contact." January 5, 2015. http://speedendurance.com/2015/01/05/triple-extension-vertical-displacement-stride-length-and-ground-contact.

Magness, Steve. "How to Run: Running with Proper Biomechanics." 2010. http://www.scienceofrunning.com/2010/08/how-to-run-running-with-proper.html.

Majumdar, Aditi, and Robert Robergs. "The Science of Speed: Determinants of Performance in the 100 M Sprint." *International Journal of Sports Science and Coaching* 6 no. 3 (2011): 479–94. doi:10.1260/1747-9541.6.3.479.

Novacheck, T. M., K. L. Siegel, S. J. Stanhope, B. R. Mason, and H. Ekstrom. "The Biomechanics of Running." *Gait & Posture* 7 no. 1 (1998): 77–95. doi:10.1016/S0966-6362(97)00038-6.

Wiemann, Klaus, and Günter Tidow. "Relative Activity of Hip and Knee Extensors in Sprinting—Implications for Training." *New Studies in Athletics* 1 no. 10 (1995): 29–49. http://richwoodstrack.com/rhs_team_area/sprints/tech_Hip Knee Extensors_wiemann.pdf.

Chapter 3

Beith, Patrick. "Running Drills for Acceleration." 2017. http://www.athletesacceleration.com/runningdrillsforacceleration.html.

Boyle, Michael. *New Functional Training for Sports,* 2nd ed. Champaign, IL: Human Kinetics, 2016.

Coleman, Eugene A., and William E. Amonette. "Pure Acceleration Is the Primary Determinant of Speed to First-Base in Major-League Baseball Game Situations." *Journal of Strength and Conditioning Research* 26 no. 6 (2012): 1455–60. doi:10.1519/JSC.0b013e3182541d56.

Contreras, Bret. "21 Questions for J. B. Morin on the Topic of Speed." The Glute Guy, 2012. https://bretcontreras.com/21-questions-for-jb-morin-on-the-topic-of-speed/.

———. "Sprint Mechanics in World-Class Athletes: A New Insight Into The Limits Of Human Locomotion." The Glute Guy, 2015. https://bretcontreras.com/sprint-mechanics-world-class-athletes-new-insight-limits-human-locomotion/.

Hunter, Joseph P., Robert N. Marshall, and Peter J. McNair. "Relationships between Ground Reaction Force Impulse and Kinematics of Sprint-Running Acceleration." *Journal of Applied Biomechanics* 21 no. 1 (2005): 31–43. http://www.ncbi.nlm.nih.gov/pubmed/16131703.

Maćkała, Krzysztof, Marek Fostiak, and Kacper Kowalski. "Selected Determinants of Acceleration in the 100m Sprint." *Journal of Human Kinetics* 45 no. 1 (2015): 135–48. doi:10.1515/hukin-2015-0014.

Mann, Ralph V., and Amber Murphy. *The Mechanics of Sprinting and Hurdling.* Las Vegas, NV: CreateSpace Independent Publishing Platform, 2015.

Maulder, Peter S., Elizabeth J. Bradshaw, and Justin Keogh. "Jump Kinetic Determinants of Sprint Acceleration Performance from Starting Blocks in Male Sprinters." *Journal of Sports Science & Medicine* 5 no. 2 (2006): 359–66. http://www.ncbi.nlm.nih.gov/pubmed/24260010.

Mero, Antti, and Paavo V. Komi. "EMG, Force, and Power Analysis of Sprint-Specific Strength Exercises." *Original Investigations Journal of Applied Biomechanics* 10 (1994): 1–13. http://fitnessforlife.org/AcuCustom/Sitename/Documents/DocumentItem/10563.pdf.

Morin, Jean-Benoît, Jean Slawinski, Sylvain Dorel, Eduardo Sàez-de-Villarreal, Antoine Couturier, Pierre Samozino, Matt Brughelli, and Giuseppe Rabita. "Acceleration Capability in Elite Sprinters and Ground Impulse: Push More, Brake Less?" *Journal of Biomechanics* 48 no. 12 (2015): 3149–54. doi:10.1016/j. jbiomech.2015.07.009.

Rabita, Giuseppi, Sylvain Dorel, Jean Slawinski, Eduardo Sàez-de-Villarreal, Antoine Couturier, Pierre Samozino, and Jean-Benoît Morin. "Sprint Mechanics in World-Class Athletes: A New Insight into the Limits of Human Locomotion." *Scandinavian Journal of Medicine & Science in Sports* 25 no. 5 (2015): 583–94. doi:10.1111/sms.12389.

Robbins, Daniel W. "Relationships Between National Football League Combine Performance Measures." *Journal of Strength and Conditioning Research* 26 no. 1 (2012): 226–31. doi:10.1519/ JSC.0b013e31821d5e1b.

Struzik, Artur, Grzegorz Konieczny, Mateusz Stawarz, Kamila Grzesik, Sławomir Winiarski, and Andrzej Rokita. "Relationship between Lower Limb Angular Kinematic Variables and the Effectiveness of Sprinting during the Acceleration Phase." *Applied Bionics and Biomechanics* vol. 2016, Article ID 7480709. doi:10.1155/2016/7480709.

Chapter 4

Cameron, Matthew L., Roger D. Adams, Chris G. Maher, David Misson. "Effect of the HamSprint Drills training programme on lower limb neuromuscular control in Australian football players." *Journal of Science and Medicine in Sport* 12 no. 1 (2009): 24–30.

Hart, Jay. "Usain Bolt, Science Of Sprinting: Case Study." 2017. http://www.thepostgame.com/ features/201107/usain-bolt-case-study-science-sprinting.

Hunter, Jayden R., Brendan J. O'Brien, Mitchell G. Mooney, Jason Berry, Warren B. Young, and Neville Down. "Repeated Sprint Training Improves Intermittent Peak Running Speed in Team-Sport Athletes." *Journal of Strength and Conditioning Research* 25 5 (2011): 1318–25. doi:10.1519/JSC.0b013e3181d85aac.

Jimson Lee. "Velocity = Contact Length / Ground Contact Time." 2011. http://speedendurance .com/2011/03/25/velocity-contact-length-ground-contact-time/.

Morin, Jean-Benoit, "Sprint Acceleration Mechanics: The Major Role of Hamstring in Horizontal Force Production." March 5, 2016. http://jbmorinsportscience.blogspot.com/2016/03/sprint-acceleration-mechanics-major.html.

Morin, Jean-Benoit, Philippe Gimenez, Pascal Edouard, Pierrick Arnal, Pedro Jimenez-Reyes, Pierre Samozino, Matt Brughelli, and Jurdan Mendiguchia. "Sprint Acceleration Mechanics: The Major Role of Hamstring in Horizontal Force Production." *Frontiers in Physiology* vol. 6: article 404 (2015):1–14. https://doi .org/10.3389/fphys.2015.00404.

Noakes, Tim. *Lore of Running.* Champaign, IL: Human Kinetics, 2003.

Performance Concepts Chat Episode 6: Ken Clark, Gait Mechanics and Running Ground Reaction Forces. 2017. *StrengthPowerSpeed.Com.* https://www.youtube.com/watch?v=Gm6pAVVFMsc.

Sacks, Andrew. "Hamstring Training for Sprinting Speed." Andrew Sacks Sports Performance, 2013. https://andrewsacksperformance.com/2013/05/11/hamstring-training-for-sprinting-speed/.

Schache, A., T. Dorn, P. Blanch, N. Brown, and M. Pandy. "Mechanics of the Human Hamstring Muscles during Sprinting." *Medicine and Science in Sports and Exercise,* vol. 44, issue 4 (2012): 647-658.

Weyand, Peter G., Rosalind F. Sandell, Danille N. L. Prime, and Matthew W. Bundle. "The Biological Limits to Running Speed Are Imposed from the Ground Up." *Journal of Applied Physiology* 108 no. 4 (2010): 950–961. http://jap.physiology.org/content/108/4/950.long.

Weyand, Peter G., Deborah B. Sternlight, Matthew J. Bellizzi, and Seth Wright. "Faster Top Running Speeds Are Achieved with Greater Ground Forces Not More Rapid Leg Movements." *Journal of Applied Physiology* 89 no. 5 (2000): 1991–1999. http://jap.physiology.org/content/89/5/1991.long.

Valle, Carl. "How Fast Can Usain Bolt Run the 40 Yard Dash?" *Freelap*. 2013. https://www.freelapusa.com/how-fast-can-usain-bolt-run-the-40-yard-dash/.

———. "Review of Al Vermeil Techniques for a Faster 40-Yard Dash." 2015. https://www.freelapusa.com/review-of-al-vermeil-techniques-for-a-faster-40-yard-dash/.

Chapter 5

Bingisser, Martin. "Special Strength: Theory and Practice." *Juggernaut*. 2017. http://www.jtsstrength.com/articles/2013/10/22/special-strength-theory-practice/.

Chumanov, Elizabeth S., Bryan C. Heiderscheit, and Darryl G. Thelen. "Hamstring Musculotendon Dynamics during Stance and Swing Phases of High-Speed Running." *Medicine and Science in Sports and Exercise* 43 no. 3 (2011): 525–32. doi:10.1249/MSS.0b013e3181f23fe8.

Contreras, Bret. "Dispelling the Glute Myth." T Nation, 2017. https://www.t-nation.com/training/dispelling-the-glute-myth.

Croisier, J. L., S. Ganteaume, J. Binet, M. Genty, and J. M. Ferret. "Strength Imbalances and Prevention of Hamstring Injury in Professional Soccer Players: A Prospective Study." *American Journal of Sports Medicine*, 36 no. 8 (2008):1469–75.

Engebretsen, Anders Hauge, Grethe Myklebust, Ingar Holme, Lars Engebretsen, and Roald Bahr. "Intrinsic Risk Factors for Hamstring Injuries Among Male Soccer Players. *The American Journal of Sports Medicine* 38 no. 6 (2010): 1147–1153. http://journals.sagepub.com/doi/abs/10.1177/0363546509358381.

Hamner, Samuel R, Ajay Seth, and Scott L. Delp. "Muscle Contributions to Propulsion and Support during Running." *Journal of Biomechanics* 43 (2010): 2709–16. doi:10.1016/j.jbiomech.2010.06.025.

Horst, Nick van der, Dirk-Wouter Smits, Jesper Petersen, Edwin A. Goedhart, and Frank J. G. Backx. "The Preventive Effect of the Nordic Hamstring Exercise on Hamstring Injuries in Amateur Soccer Players." *The American Journal of Sports Medicine* 43 no. 6 (2015): 1316–23. doi:10.1177/0363546515574057.

Kraemer, R., and K. Knobloch. "A Soccer-Specific Balance Training Program for Hamstring Muscle and Patellar and Achilles Tendon Injuries: An Intervention Study in Premier League Female Soccer." *The American Journal of Sports Medicine* 37 no. 7 (2009): 1384–93. doi:10.1177/0363546509333012.

Kyröläinen, Heikki, Janne Avela, and Paavo V. Komi. "Changes in muscle activity with increasing running speed." *Journal of Sports Sciences*, 23 no. 10 (2005): 1101–1109.

Liu, Hui, William E. Garrett, and Claude T. Moorman. 2012. "Injury Rate, Mechanism, and Risk Factors of Hamstring Strain Injuries in Sports: A Review of the Literature." Journal of Sport and Health Science 1 no. 2 (2012): 92–101. doi:10.1016/j.jshs.2012.07.003.

Liu, Yu, Yuliang Sun, Wenfei Zhu, and Jiabin Yu. "The Late Swing and Early Stance of Sprinting Are Most Hazardous for Hamstring Injuries." *Journal of Sport and Health Science* 6 no. 2 (2017): 133–136. doi:10.1016/j.jshs.2017.01.011.

Magness, Steve. "The Most Important Information You Will Ever Read about Running Form: Passive vs. Active." 2011. http://www.scienceofrunning.com/2011/04/most-important-information-you-will.html.

Mann, Ralph, and Paul Sprague. "A Kinetic Analysis of the Ground Leg During Sprint Running." *Research Quarterly for Exercise and Sport* 51 vol. 2 (1980): 334–48. doi:10.1080/02701367.1980.10605202.

Munn, J., R. D. Herbert, and S. C. Gandevia. "Contralateral Effects of Unilateral Resistance Training: A Meta-Analysis." *Journal of Applied Physiology* 96 no. 5 (2004): 1861–1866. http://jap.physiology.org/content/96/5/1861.

Nicola, Terry L., and David J. Jewison. "The Anatomy and Biomechanics of Running." *Clinics in Sports Medicine* 31 vol. 2 (2012): 187–201. doi:10.1016/j.csm.2011.10.001.

Panariello, Robert A. "Four Reasons Why Athletes Must Sprint–Bret Contreras." 2015. https://bretcontreras.com/four-reasons-why-athletes-must-sprint/.

Petersen, Jesper, Kristian Thorborg, Michael Bachmann Nielsen, Esben Budtz-Jørgensen, and Per Hölmich. "Preventive Effect of Eccentric Training on Acute Hamstring Injuries in Men's Soccer." *The American Journal of Sports Medicine* 39 no. 11 (2011): 2296–2303. doi:10.1177/0363546511419277.

Schuermans, Joke, Lieven Danneels, Damien Van Tiggelen, Tanneke Palmans, and Erik Witvrouw. "Proximal Neuromuscular Control Protects Against Hamstring Injuries in Male Soccer Players: A Prospective Study With Electromyography Time-Series Analysis During Maximal Sprinting." *The American Journal of Sports Medicine* 45 no. 6 (2017): 1315–25. doi:10.1177/0363546516687750.

Sherry, Marc A., and Thomas M. Best. "A Comparison of 2 Rehabilitation Programs in the Treatment of Acute Hamstring Strains." *Journal of Orthopedic & Sports Physical Therapy* 34 (2004): 116–25. http://www.uwhealth.org/files/uwhealth/docs/pdf3/sportsrehab_sherry.pdf.

Silder, Amy, Darryl G. Thelen, and Bryan C. Heiderscheit. "Effects of Prior Hamstring Strain Injury on Strength, Flexibility, and Running Mechanics." *Clinical Biomechanics* 25 no. 7 (2010): 681–86. doi:10.1016/j.clinbiomech.2010.04.015.

Sugiura, Y., T. Saito, K. Sakuraba, K. Sakuma, and E. Suzuki. "Strength Deficits Identified With Concentric Action of the Hip Extensors and Eccentric Action of the Hamstrings Predispose to Hamstring Injury in Elite Sprinters." *Journal of Orthopaedic & Sports Physical Therapy*, vol. 38, no. 8 (2008): 457–464.

Chapter 6

Chaouachi, Anis, Moktar Chtara, Raouf Hammami, Hichem Chtara, Olfa Turki, and Carlo Castagna. "Multidirectional Sprints and Small-Sided Games Training Effect on Agility and Change of Direction Abilities in Youth Soccer." *Journal of Strength and Conditioning Research* 28 no. 11 (2014): 3121–27. doi:10.1519/JSC.0000000000000505.

Han, Jia, Gordon Waddington, Judith Anson, and Roger Adams. "Level of Competitive Success Achieved by Elite Athletes and Multi-Joint Proprioceptive Ability." *Journal of Science and Medicine in Sport* 18 no. 1 (2015): 77–81. doi:10.1016/j.jsams.2013.11.013.

Ibrahim, Victor, Zinovy Meyler, and Andre Panagos. "ACSM Current Comment." *American College of Sports Medicine*. 2017. http://www.shapeamerica.org/publications/resources/teachingtools/coachtoolbox/upload/Ankle-Sprains-and-the-Athlete.pdf.

Keown, Tim. "Speed Freaks." *ESPN*. 2012. http://www.espn.com/espn/magazine/archives/news/story?page=magazine-20020527-article37.

McHugh, M., T. Tyler, M. Mirabella, M. Mullaney., and S. Nicholas. "The Effectiveness of a Balance Training Intervention in Reducing the Incidence of Noncontact Ankle Sprains in High School Football Players." *American Journal of Sports Medicine*, 35 no. 8 (2007): 1289–1294. doi:10:1177/0363546507300059.

Milanović, Zoran, Goran Sporiš, Nebojša Trajković, Nic James, and Krešimir Samija. "Effects of a 12 Week SAQ Training Programme on Agility with and without the Ball among Young Soccer Players." *Journal of Sports Science & Medicine* 12 no. 1 (2013): 97–103. http://www.ncbi.nlm.nih.gov/pubmed/24149731.

Oliveira, Anderson Souza, Priscila Brito Silva, Morten Enemark Lund, Leonardo Gizzi, Dario Farina, and Uwe Gustav Kersting. "Effects of Perturbations to Balance on Neuromechanics of Fast Changes in Direction during Locomotion." Ed. Alejandro Lucia. *PLOS ONE* 8 no. 3 (2013): e59029. doi:10.1371/journal.pone.0059029.

Paul, Darren, Tim Gabbett, and George Nassis. "Agility in Team Sports: Testing, Training and Factors Affecting Performance." *Sports Medicine*. 46 no. 3 (2015): 421-442. doi: 10.1007/s40279-015-0428-2.

Ricotti, Leonardo. "Static and Dynamic Balance in Young Athletes." *Journal of Human Sport & Exercise* 6 no. 4 (2011): 616–28. doi:10.4100/jhse.2011.64.05.

Serpell B. G., W. B. Young, M., and Ford M. "Are the Perceptual and Decision-Making Components of Agility Trainable? A Preliminary Investigation." *Journal of Strength Conditioning Research* 25 no. 5 (2011): 1240–8.

Sheppard, J. M., and W. B. Young. "Agility Literature Review: Classifications, Training and Testing." *Journal of Sports Sciences* 24 no. 9 (2006): 919–32. doi:10.1080/02640410500457109.

Sheppard, J. M., W. B. Young, T. L. A. Doyle, T. A. Sheppard., R. U. Newton. "An Evaluation of a New Test of Reactive Agility and its Relationship to Sprint Speed and Change of Direction Speed." *Journal of Science and Medicine in Sport* vol. 9 (2006): 342–349.

Chapter 7

Balsalobre-Fernández, Carlos, Jordan Santos-Concejero, and Gerasimos V. Grivas. "Effects of Strength Training on Running Economy in Highly Trained Runners." *Journal of Strength and Conditioning Research* 30 no. 8 (2016): 2361–68. doi:10.1519/JSC.0000000000001316.

Iaia, F. Marcello, Matteo Fiorenza, Enrico Perri, Giampietro Alberti, Grégoire P. Millet, and Jens Bangsbo. "The Effect of Two Speed Endurance Training Regimes on Performance of Soccer Players." Ed. Oyvind Sandbakk. *PLOS ONE* 10 no. 9 (2015): e0138096. doi:10.1371/journal.pone.0138096.

Ross, A., and M. Leveritt. "Long-Term Metabolic and Skeletal Muscle Adaptations to Short-Sprint Training: Implications for Sprint Training and Tapering." *Sports Medicine (Auckland, N.Z.)* 31 vol. 15 (2001): 1063–82. http://www.ncbi.nlm.nih.gov/pubmed/11735686.

Chapter 8

American Academy of Sleep Medicine. "Extra Sleep Improves Athletic Performance." *ScienceDaily*. June 10, 2008. www.sciencedaily.com/releases/2008/06/080609071106.htm

Dalleck, Lance C. "The Science of Post-Exercise Recovery." *American Council on Exercise*. 2016. https://acewebcontent.azureedge.net/SAP-Reports/Post-Exercise_Recovery_SAP_Reports.pdf.

Fitzpatrick, Jane, Max Bulsara, and Ming H. Zheng. 2017. "The Effectiveness of Platelet-Rich Plasma in the Treatment of Tendinopathy: A Meta-Analysis of Randomized Controlled Clinical Trials." *The American Journal of Sports Medicine* 45 no. 1 (2016): 226–33. doi:10.1177/0363546516643716.

Gambetta, Vernon. "Defining Supercompensation Training." *Human Kinetics.* 2007. http://www.humankinetics.com/excerpts/excerpts/defining-supercompensation-training.

Ingraham, Paul. "Does Chiropractic Work?" *PainScience.com,* 2016. https://www.painscience.com/articles/does-chiropractic-work.php.

Jenkins, Sally. "Peyton Manning on His Neck Surgeries Rehab—and How He Almost Didn't Make It Back." *The Washington Post,* October 21, 2013. https://www.washingtonpost.com/sports/redskins/peyton-manning-on-his-neck-surgeries-rehab--and-how-he-almost-didnt-make-it-back/2013/10/21/8e3b5ca6-3a55-11e3-b7ba-503fb5822c3e_story.html.

Khoshbin, Amir, Timothy Leroux, David Wasserstein, Paul Marks, John Theodoropoulos, Darrell Ogilvie-Harris, Rajiv Ganhi, Kirat Takhar, Grant Lum, and Jaskarndip Chahal. "The Efficacy of Platelet-Rich Plasma in the Treatment of Symptomatic Knee Osteoarthritis: A Systematic Review with Quantitative Synthesis." *Arthroscopy: The Journal of Arthroscopic & Related Surgery.* 29, no. 12 (2013): 2037-2048.

MacMillan, Amanda. "How Do Pro Athletes Recover So Quickly?" *Outside Online,* 2015. https://www.outsideonline.com/1786196/how-do-pro-athletes-recover-so-quickly.

Magill, Pete. "Inflammation: Friend or Foe?" *Running Times.* November 1, 2010. https://www.runnersworld.com/website-only/inflammation-friend-or-foe.

Magill, Pete, Melissa Breyer, and Thomas Schwartz. *Build Your Running Body: A Total-Body Fitness Plan for All Distance Runners, from Milers to Ultramarathoners.* New York: The Experiment, 2014.

Mah, Cheri D., Kenneth E. Mah, Eric J. Kezirian, and William C. Dement. "The Effects of Sleep Extension on the Athletic Performance of Collegiate Basketball Players." *Sleep* 34 no. 7 (2011): 943–50. doi:10.5665/SLEEP.1132.

Mostafavifar, Mehran, Jess Wertz, and James Borchers. "A Systematic Review of the Effectiveness of Kinesio Taping for Musculoskeletal Injury." *The Physician and Sportsmedicine* 40 no. 4 (2012): 33–40. doi:10.3810/psm.2012.11.1986.

Parreira, Patricia do Carmo Silva, Lucola da Cunha Menezes Costa, Luiz Carlos Hespanhol Junior, Alexandre Dias Lopes, and Leonardo Oliveira Pena Costa. "Current Evidence Does Not Support the Use of Kinesio Taping in Clinical Practice: A Systematic Review." *Journal of Physiotherapy* 60 no. 1 (2014): 31–39. doi:10.1016/j.jphys.2013.12.008.

Petrofsky, Jerrold Scott, Michael Laymon, and Haneul Lee. "Effect of Heat and Cold on Tendon Flexibility and Force to Flex the Human Knee." *Medical Science Monitor: International Medical Journal of Experimental and Clinical Research* 19 (2013): 661–667.

Roberts, Llion A., Truls Raastad, James F. Markworth, Vandre C. Figueiredo, Ingrid M. Egner, Anthony Shield, David Cameron-Smith, Jeff S. Coombes, and Jonathan M. Peake. "Post-Exercise Cold Water Immersion Attenuates Acute Anabolic Signalling and Long-Term Adaptations in Muscle to Strength Training." *The Journal of Physiology* 593 no. 18 (2015): 4285–4301. doi:10.1113/JP270570.

Rubinstein, S. M., C. B. Terwee, W. J. J. Assendelft, M. R. de Boer, and M. W. van Tulder. "Spinal manipulative therapy for acute low-back pain." *Cochrane Database of Systematic Reviews* Issue 9, Article. No.: CD008880. 2012. doi: 10.1002/14651858.CD008880.pub2.

"Study: Platelet-Rich Plasma for Tendinopathy? Researchers See Promise." *PT in Motion News,* 2017. http://www.apta.org/PTinMotion/News/2017/6/7/PRPForTendinopathy/.

Tucker, Ross, Jonathan Dugas, and Matt Fitzgerald. *The Runner's Body: How the Latest Exercise Science Can Help You Run Stronger, Longer, and Faster.* Emmaus, PA: Rodale, 2009.

Vingren, Jakob L, David W. Hill, Harsh Buddhadev, and Anthony Duplanty. "Postresistance Exercise Ethanol Ingestion and Acute Testosterone Bioavailability." *Medicine & Science in Sports & Exercise* 45 no. 9 (2013): 1825–32. doi:10.1249/MSS.0b013e31828d3767.

Zurawlew, M. J., N. P. Walsh, M. B. Fortes, and C. Potter. "Post-Exercise Hot Water Immersion Induces Heat Acclimation and Improves Endurance Exercise Performance in the Heat." *Scandinavian Journal of Medicine & Science in Sports* 26 no. 7 (2016): 745–54. doi:10.1111/sms.12638.

Chapter 9

Marques, M., T. Gabbett, D. Marinho, A. Blazevich, A. Sousa, R. van den Tillaar, and M. Izquierdo. "Influence of Strength, Sprint Running, and Combined Strength and Sprint Running Training on Short Sprint Performance in Young Adults." *International Journal of Sports Medicine* 36 no. 10 (2015): 789–95. doi:10.1055/s-0035-1547284.

Rhea, M., J. Kenn, M. Peterson, et al. "Joint-Angle Specific Strength Adaptations Influence Improvements in Power in Highly Trained Athletes." *Human Movement,* 17 no. 1 (2016): 43–49. doi:10.1515/humo-2016-0006.

ABOUT THE CONTRIBUTORS

Diana Hernandez

Diana Hernandez is the photographer for the books *Build Your Running Body* and *The Born Again Runner*. Her work has appeared in *Runner's World, Competitor*, and *Running Times*, as well as on websites such as *The Huffington Post* and *Outside*. When not shooting fitness and action photography, Hernandez is a 9th grade biology teacher for Santee Education Complex in Los Angeles, CA.

Sean Magill

Sean Magill utilized SpeedRunner training to earn first team all-league honors in high school football and track, trained under internationally acclaimed strength coach Robert dos Remedios during college football, and will receive his BS in human physiology from the University of Oregon in 2018. He helped formulate and execute the SpeedRunner study in 2016 that verified SpeedRunner performance gains.

Eric Dixon

Eric Dixon is the director for USA Track & Field's Level 1 Schools for Coaches in Southern California, a spokesperson for USATF's "Win with Integrity Program," and the former head sprint coach for the US Air Force Wounded Warrior track team. He has designed speed and agility programs for the AYSO Coaches Training Camp, Lifeletics (baseball), and Tachyon Track Club, among others.

INDEX

Italicized page numbers indicate a table or chart.

ABOUT THE AUTHOR

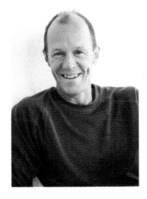

Pete Magill is the lead author of the book *Build Your Running Body*, author of *The Born Again Runner*, and a former senior writer and columnist for *Running Times* magazine, where his popular "Performance Page" column tracked the latest advances in exercise physiology. A five-time USA Masters Cross Country Runner of the Year, two-time USA age group runner of the year, and three-time USA masters track and field age group athlete of the year, Magill holds multiple American and world age-group records and has led his clubs to 19 national championships in cross country and road racing. He's a high school sprint coach, running coach for the California Triathlon Club, and masters coach for the Cal Coast Track Club, as well as co-owner of SpeedRunner LLC and head instructor for all Southern California SpeedRunner training and instructor certification programs. He lives in South Pasadena, California.

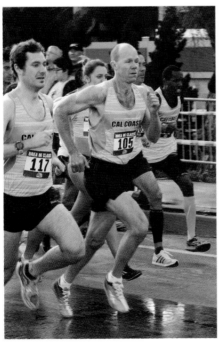